Children with
Prenatal Alcohol and/or
Other Drug Exposure

Children with Prenatal Alcohol and/or Other Drug Exposure:

Weighing the Risks of Adoption

Susan B. Edelstein

with contributions from

Judy Howard, Rachelle Tyler,
Gloria Waldinger, & Annette Moore

CWLA Press • Washington, DC

CWLA Press is an imprint of the Child Welfare League of America.

© 1995 by the Child Welfare League of America, Inc.

CHILD WELFARE LEAGUE OF AMERICA, INC.
440 First Street, NW, Suite 310, Washington, DC 20001-2085

CURRENT PRINTING (last digit)
10 9 8 7 6 5 4 3 2 1

Cover design by Ed Zielinski
Text design by Jennifer M. Canfield

Printed in the United States of America

ISBN # 0–87868–630–4

*This book is dedicated
to the memory of my father,
Joseph Sacks.*

Contents

Acknowledgments

As the principal author, I owe a debt of gratitude to many people—friends, clients, colleagues, mentors, and contributing authors—who added to this volume over time and in many ways.

It is an honor to have worked with children, parents, and families for over 27 years. I have approached this work from several vantage points—I began my professional career in child protective services, then specialized in adoption, and, in 1979, expanded my focus into health care. At UCLA Medical Center, I have been a member of several interdisciplinary teams involved in the issues surrounding child abuse and neglect, maternal-child health, chemical dependency, and child development. To have been engaged for so many years in work that has abounded in challenges, meaning, opportunities, and variety has truly been a privilege. I want to extend a special thanks to all of the clients—children as well as adults—from whom I have learned so much by sharing in their lives, their troubles, their strengths, and their triumphs.

During my years with the Los Angeles County Department of Adoptions, I benefited greatly from the mentorship, dedication, and vision of many outstanding professionals. Matille Rufrano, Mary Connery, Audrey Rinker, Dale Weiss, Blossom Nishime, and Carolyn Epling all possessed wisdom that was well beyond their times, and I reflect frequently on the thoughtfulness and skill they brought to every case discussion.

At UCLA Medical Center, I have enjoyed the opportunity and privilege of working with highly talented professionals from a number of disciplines within the University and from the broader community as well.

I am deeply grateful for the mentorship of Judy Howard, M.D., whose creativity, resourcefulness, and energy have provided me with a valuable example. Additionally, her pioneering advocacy in behalf of children with prenatal substance exposure and her strong belief in early intervention, interdisciplinary collaboration, and community service have been enormously important to me as I conceptualized this book.

Vickie Kropenske, P.H.N., M.S.N., with her dedication to serving vulnerable families, her high standards, and her exemplary skills, has been a constant source of inspiration. I learn from her daily.

For over a decade, I have shared ideas, projects, and clients with Rachelle Tyler, M.D. Her humor, balanced ideas, and ongoing deep interest in working with child welfare practitioners and clients is truly heartening and a source of strength for me and all with whom she interacts.

Annette Moore, M.A., has provided invaluable support, advice, friendship, and editorial assistance in the preparation of this manuscript. When it was only an idea, she recognized the importance of writing this book. With her hard work, encouragement, and perseverance, she contributed significantly to making this long-term professional aspiration a reality.

I also want to thank Gloria Waldinger, D.S.W., who recruited me to serve as coordinator of the Suspected Child Abuse and Neglect (SCAN) Team at UCLA Medical Center, where I learned important lessons about teamwork. Without that experience, this book would not have been written. Throughout the years, I have repeatedly drawn upon Gloria's expertise. She also provided feedback in the preparation of this manuscript.

Finally, Mary Ann Skelton, M.A., and Kathy McTaggart, M.F.C.C.—who are adoptive parents as well as skilled practitioners—have influenced me beyond measure by their resilience, courage, struggles, and strengths.

The individual and collective skill, wisdom, and dedication of many others have influenced my thinking and contributed to my personal and professional growth over the years I have worked at

UCLA Medical Center. The physicians—Cheryl Breitenbach-Wickham, Claudia Wang, M. Lynn Yonekura, and Arthur H. Parmelee; the social workers—Mary Beth Sorensen, Charles L. Edwards, Brenda Martin, Nancy Hayes, and Rose Monteiro; the nurses—Bette Billet, Maxyne Strunin, Mary Troutman, Jeanne Smart, Karen Fond, Debi Roberts, and Marty Jessup; the psychologists—Morris Paulson, Leila Beckwith, and Michael Espinosa; the attorneys—James Holst, Karen DuBois, Robert Goldstein, and Virginia Weisz; a very special volunteer—Joann Solov; and administrative support staff—Ellen Silk, Maria Gonzalez, and Rosa Prado, all taught me the value of synergy and interdisciplinary collaboration.

Special thanks are also due to the individuals who offered their personal encouragement and support—Dwight and Grace Warren, Clare Lake, Jean Barrett, and William Matchett—and to Donna Haas, who reviewed the manuscript and offered helpful advice.

I am deeply grateful for the patience, cooperation, and unfailing support of my husband, Jerry, and our daughter, Robin. They consistently believed in the importance of this "labor of love" and in my ability to articulate what needed to be written on this important topic.

In addition, thanks are owed to Jean McIntosh, who pointed me in the direction of the Child Welfare League of America when I approached her about writing on adoption of children with prenatal substance exposure, and to Ann Sullivan of CWLA, who knew immediately that this was a book that had to be written, and very soon. Finally, I want to express my appreciation for the perseverance, skill, and insights of my editor, Carl Schoenberg, who helped bring a clear form to this work.

Susan B. Edelstein

Introduction

Adoption is increasingly recognized as a dynamic, ongoing, lifelong
process for all parties involved. [Sorich & Siebert 1982: 216]

This book offers suggestions, recommendations, and food for thought
for preparing, counseling, and working over the long term with
prospective adoptive parents who are considering adopting an infant or child who has been exposed prenatally to alcohol and/or
other drugs. For the past 12 years, the authors' multidisciplinary,
hospital-based team of pediatricians, social workers, public health
nurses, and child development specialists has worked on a wide
range of clinical service, research, and training projects serving
hundreds of biological parents, kinship caregivers, foster parents,
adoptive parents, and service providers with regard to the special
needs of children exposed prenatally to alcohol and/or drugs, as
well as the special needs of their caregivers.

Significant gaps in information and services have come to our
attention over the years. Many relate to the issues faced by adoption
workers and prospective adoptive parents concerning infants and
children whose biological parents have problems related to substance abuse. The literature on adoption overall is considerable,
including a significant amount of information about the adoption of
children who have special needs and a growing but still limited body
of information about children who were exposed prenatally to alcohol and/or other drugs. Information about preadoption counseling
for individuals who are considering adopting a child with prenatal
substance exposure, however, is meager.

Over the years, the authors have received countless urgent phone calls from prospective adoptive parents wanting help in deciding whether to adopt a child who was exposed prenatally to alcohol and/or other drugs. In many cases, these persons have had to make their decisions very quickly, as the baby had just been born and was awaiting placement in an adoptive home. In other instances, the biological mother was still pregnant, and prospective adoptive parents were wondering about potential risks in terms of short- and long-term outcomes for the child. In still other situations, foster parents or kinship caregivers who already had a young child in their home had many questions about the child's future.

The decision to adopt a child should be thoughtfully made, and considerable reflection, discussion, and gathering of information should precede it. The same is true of the decision to adopt a child with prenatal substance exposure. This decision has lifelong implications for the child, the biological parents, and the adoptive family, and should be made only after thorough consideration of the risks and challenges—as well as the potentials and opportunities—involved. It is not a conclusion to be reached on the basis of a telephone conversation or a meeting with an expert regarding his or her research or clinical impressions concerning substance exposure and children to date, or after reading a few articles or media accounts.

In addition to examining the risks and potentials involved for children with prenatal substance exposure, the professional and the individual or couple considering adoption need to examine the abilities, skills, and attitudes of the prospective parents that will contribute toward successful adoption of a child who has been exposed prenatally to alcohol and/or other drugs. Not all well-functioning couples or individuals have the particular capabilities needed to raise an adopted child successfully [Katz 1980], much less an adopted child with prenatal substance exposure. Thus, it is important to explore the special aspects of adoptive parenthood of a child who has been exposed prenatally to alcohol and/or other drugs.

Background: Prenatal Substance Abuse

The drug epidemic that began in the early 1980s has had a devastating effect on families and on children in this country. Substance abuse has weakened the fabric of our families—when parents are in its clutches, the quest for drugs often takes precedence over their children's needs and care. Parental abuse of alcohol and/or other drugs has been associated with an increased incidence of child abuse and neglect, an increase in out-of-home placement of children, and a growing number of children born with in-utero alcohol and/or other drug exposure. Because chemical dependency complicates family reunification efforts, and because the rates of successful drug treatment for chronically addicted individuals are not heartening [Besharov 1989], a growing number of infants and children with prenatal alcohol and/or other drug exposure are in need of permanent homes. Adoption is one means of providing those homes.

Although available data are imprecise at best, it is estimated that over 4.8 million women of childbearing age use illicit drugs [Johnson 1992]. The number of infants born each year with prenatal exposure to alcohol and/or other drugs lies somewhere between 554,000 and 739,000 [Gomby & Shiono 1991]. Even at the low end of this estimate, a substance-exposed infant is born more frequently than every 90 seconds [Schipper 1991]. A recent study conducted by researchers at the School of Public Health at the University of California, Berkeley, found that the number of maternity patients at California hospitals in 1992 who had used drugs (legal or illegal, not including tobacco) or alcohol within several days of delivery was 11.35%—one of every nine women [Los Angeles County Department of Health Services, Alcohol & Drug Program Administration 1993; Vega et al. 1993]. Further, these estimates are considered conservative because they were based on urine toxicology screens, which can detect only recent substance use. The actual rates of substance abuse during pregnancy are probably even higher.

Besides the biological risk that prenatal alcohol and/or other drug exposure presents to the fetus, infant, and child, parents who abuse substances are at increased risk of abusing and/or neglecting their children [Bays 1990; Famularo et al. 1992; Mayer & Black 1977; Regan et al. 1987]. The sharp increase in the number of substance-affected families with children and the escalating number of children with prenatal drug exposure have contributed substantially to the rising number of children in out-of-home placements in this country [Feig 1990; American Public Welfare Association 1991]. Child abuse and neglect reports increased by 100% between 1982 and 1992, and the number of children living outside their own homes also rose at an alarming rate during this same period [Child Welfare League of America 1994]. In 1985, 276,000 children were in out-of-home care. By 1992, the number had risen to 429,000 [Tatara 1990, 1993]. If this trend continues, a projected 553,600 children will be in out-of-home placements in the U.S. in 1995 [Select Committee on Children, Youth and Families 1990].

Adoption of Children with Prenatal Substance Exposure

Although achieving family reunification is still the goal for child welfare professionals working with substance-abusing parents [American Public Welfare Association 1991], many children of substance-abusing parents (including many children who were exposed prenatally to alcohol and/or other drugs) require placement with relatives, foster parents, or, eventually, adoptive parents. Substance abuse is a long-term, chronic condition that is difficult to treat. Studies have shown that suitable treatment resources often are unavailable and that reunification with biological parents occurs only half as frequently in situations involving parental substance abuse as in situations where parental abuse of alcohol and/or other drugs is not a factor [Walker 1994].

Unless children who cannot be reunified with their biological parents are placed permanently, be it by guardianship or adoption, their risk status for lifelong developmental and/or emotional complications is likely to be heightened due to multiple placements and the almost inevitably deleterious sequelae of inconsistent caregiving. Kinship care should be used when possible if children must be removed permanently from their biological parents [American Public Welfare Association 1991]. When relatives are unavailable, adoptive placement with well-prepared, nonrelated persons, if possible from the same cultural background, is critical if the children are to achieve security and stability [Child Welfare League of America 1992].

Throughout the U.S., children with prenatal alcohol and/or other drug exposure represent a growing proportion of the larger population of children who are in need of permanency. Many of these children will attain permanency through adoption. According to reports from adoptive parents in California from mid-1988 to mid-1989, 25% of adopted children had been exposed prenatally to alcohol and/or other drugs [Barth 1991]; estimates from professionals working daily in the field are even higher. Because kinship caregivers as well as nonrelated adults are increasingly becoming adoptive parents of infants who were exposed prenatally to alcohol and/or drugs, or are at least considering the possibility of adopting children who have such exposure, and because it is difficult to find a prospective adoptive child about whom one can be sure there has been no prenatal substance exposure, the breadth and variety of factors likely to be involved in these adoptions must be examined thoroughly.

Summary

The information in this book is intended primarily to assist professionals in guiding nonrelated prospective adoptive parents considering adoption of substance-exposed infants through the issues they should consider at this important juncture in their lives. Many of the same issues, however, are also pertinent for relatives who are considering adoption, although with critical variations that lie beyond the scope of this book.

Infants and children exposed to substances prenatally come into adoption in a variety of ways. In some instances, biological parents may voluntarily relinquish an infant shortly after birth to a public or private agency for adoption, or may arrange an independent adoption. In other cases, biological parents may relinquish relatively older children. Other substance-exposed children become available for adoption when parental rights are terminated by the courts because of the biological parents' inability to provide a safe and nurturing home for their children and the children's need for a permanent plan.

Some children who have been made available for adoption at a relatively later point in life, whether through parental relinquishment or court action, may have experienced nurturing, stable environments and may, in fact, be adopted by the same people with whom they have been living and with whom they have developed loving ties. Other children, however, in an all-too-common scenario, may have experienced severe deprivation in the form of prolonged hospitalizations or child abuse and neglect. Still others may have problems attendant to multiple placements with kinship caregivers, foster parents, or adoptive parents, or placement in group settings. These situations and their serious and complex implications are not separated out in this book from the effects of prenatal substance exposure itself. Professionals do have access, however, to a growing body of knowledge about the sequelae of child abuse and neglect and parental deprivation, and many are using this expertise in their work with families who are adopting relatively older children.

Additionally, for practical intervention strategies that have been found to be helpful in working directly with infants, toddlers, and older children who have been exposed prenatally to drugs, the reader is referred to a growing and readily available literature describing such useful interventions [Healey 1993; Kleinfeld & Wescott 1993; Kropenske et al. 1994a, 1994b; Lecca & Watts 1993; Los Angeles Unified School District 1989; Smith et al. 1995; Tyler 1992].

The clinical considerations presented in this book are not the result of research. Rather, they are descriptions of clinical findings, reflections, and observations that have been integrated with theories of adoption, chemical dependency, and child development. Many of these concepts represent educated guesses; they are not intended to provide neat, cookbook guidelines. Both now and in the future, empirical research is acutely needed to determine whether these or other considerations are truly of value in helping prospective adoptive parents and the professionals with whom they work explore the interests, knowledge, perspectives, and abilities that enable parents to provide effective and meaningful care for children exposed prenatally to drugs.

Based on the extensive experience of a range of professionals who have worked with substance-affected families as well as on the experience of a variety of individuals—both professionals and lay persons—who have been involved in the adoption process, this book provides a foundation for in-depth thinking and discussion for adoption practitioners. Basic material about general adoption theory has also been included to make the book useful for the broad range of professionals who may not be familiar with adoption literature overall. As a resource for service providers, the book can also indirectly help families and others in the adoption arena.

Chapter One discusses the limitations of existing research on prenatal exposure to alcohol and/or other drugs, the resulting difficulties in predicting outcomes for individual children, and the impediments to adopting children exposed prenatally to drugs. It also deals with the lack of integration among the components of chemical dependency, prenatal substance exposure, and adoption, and the resulting gap in knowledge about how best to prepare prospective applicants for adoption of children with prenatal drug exposure. Chapter Two describes what is known about the health and development of infants and children who were exposed to alcohol and/or other drugs in utero. Chapters Three and Four discuss the unique considerations for prospective adoptive parents who are contemplating adoption of these special children—including perspectives on origins, loss, uncertainty, and open adoption, as well as on approaching the adoption from a risk-and-protective-factors standpoint rather than a deficit perspective.

Finally, Chapter Five outlines recommendations emerging from the preceding material. It is almost impossible to ponder preadoption counseling in this special arena without also considering the types of postadoption services that will be necessary for these children and families. The two areas are closely intertwined. On the one hand, prospective adoptive parents need information and anticipatory guidance to alert them to be open and receptive to certain services, if and when these are indicated, that will help support their children and their families in the future. On the other hand, these services must be available if we are to maximize the prospect for successful adoption of an individual child.

References

American Public Welfare Association. (1991). *Guiding principles for working with substance-abusing families and drug-exposed children: The child welfare response*. Recommendations of the National Association of Public Child Welfare Administrators, approved by the Executive Committee of the National Council of State Human Services Administrators. Washington, DC: American Public Welfare Association.

Barth, R. P. (1991). Adoption of drug-exposed children. *Children and Youth Services Review, 13*, 323–342.

Bays, J. (1990). Substance abuse and child abuse: Impact of addiction on the child. *Pediatric Clinics of North America, 37*, 881–904.

Besharov, D. J. (1989). The children of crack: Will we protect them? *Public Welfare, 47*(4), 6–11.

Child Welfare League of America. (1992). *Children at the front: A different view of the war on alcohol and drugs. Final report and recommendations of the CWLA North American Commission on Chemical Dependency and Child Welfare.* Washington, DC: Author.

Child Welfare League of America. (1994). *Kinship care: A natural bridge.* Washington, DC: Author.

Famularo, R., Kinscherff, R., & Fenton, T. (1992). Parental substance abuse and the nature of child maltreatment. *Child Abuse & Neglect, 16,* 475–483.

Feig, L. (1990, August). *Drug-exposed infants and children: Service needs and policy questions.* Washington, DC: U.S. Department of Health and Human Services, Office of the Assistant Secretary for Planning and Evaluation (unpublished report).

Gomby, D., & Shiono, P. (1991). Estimating the number of substance-exposed infants. *The Future of Children, 1*(1), 17.

Healey, T. (199). Intervention strategies in children exposed prenatally to drugs...a continuum birth through school age. *The Clearinghouse for Drug Exposed Children Newsletter, 4*(3), 1–3, 6.

Johnson, E. M. (1992). Foreword. In S. L. Quinton, S. A. Johnson, E. M. Johnson, R. W. Denniston, & K. L. Augustson (Eds.), *Identifying the needs of drug-affected children: Public policy issues* (pp. iii–iv). OSAP prevention monograph 11. Rockville, MD: Office for Substance Abuse Prevention, U.S. Department of Health and Human Services (OSAP prevention monograph 11, DHHS publication number (ADM) 92–1814).

Katz, L. (1980). Adoption counseling as a preventive mental health specialty. *Child Welfare, 59,* 161–167.

Kleinfeld, J., & Wescott, S. (1993). *Fantastic Antone succeeds: Experiences in educating children with Fetal Alcohol Syndrome.* Fairbanks, AK: University of Alaska Press.

Kropenske, V., Breitenbach, C., Edelstein, S. B., Howard, J., McTaggart, K. K., Moore, A., Sorensen, M. B., Tyler, R., & Weisz, V. (1994a). *Supporting substance-abusing families: A technical assistance manual for the Head Start management team.* Washington, DC: U.S. Department of Health and Human Services, Administration for Children and Families, Administration for Children, Youth and Families, Head Start Bureau (U.S. Government Printing Office 1994–515–032–03031).

Kropenske, V., & Howard, J., with Breitenbach, C., Dembo, R., Edelstein, S. B., McTaggart, K., Moore, A., Sorensen, M. B., & Weisz, V. (1994b). *Protecting children in substance-abusing families.* Washington, DC: U.S.

Department of Health and Human Services/National Center on Child Abuse and Neglect (User manual series).

Lecca, P. J., & Watts, T. D. (1993). *Preschoolers and substance abuse: Strategies for prevention and intervention.* New York: The Haworth Press, Inc.

Los Angeles County Department of Health Services, Alcohol & Drug Program Administration. (1993). *Fact sheet: State of California—Perinatal substance exposure study.* Los Angeles: Author.

Los Angeles Unified School District. (1989). *Today's challenge: Teaching strategies for working with young children prenatally exposed to drugs/ alcohol, July 1989.* Los Angeles: Los Angeles Unified School District, Division of Special Education, Prenatally Exposed to Drugs Program.

Mayer, J., & Black, R. (1977). Child abuse and neglect in families with an alcohol or opiate addicted parent. *Child Abuse & Neglect, 1,* 85–98.

Regan, D. O., Ehrlich, S. M., & Finnegan, L. P. (1987). Infants of drug addicts: At risk for child abuse, neglect, and placement in foster care. *Neurotoxicology and Teratology, 9,* 315–319.

Schipper, W. (1991, July 30). *Testimony before the U.S. House of Representatives Select Committee on Narcotics Abuse and Control.*

Smith, G. H., Coles, C. D., Poulsen, M. K., & Cole, C. K. (1995). *Children, families, and substance abuse: Challenges for changing educational and social outcomes.* Baltimore: Paul H. Brookes Publishing Co.

Sorich, C. J., & Siebert, R. (1982). Toward humanizing adoption. *Child Welfare, 61,* 207–16.

Tatara, T. (1990). *Children of substance-abusing/alcoholic parents referred to the public child welfare system: Summaries of key statistical data obtained from states.* Washington, DC: American Public Welfare Association.

Tatara, T. (1993, January 19). Personal communication re FY 1991 data.

Tyler, R. (1992). Prenatal drug exposure: An overview of associated problems and intervention strategies. *Phi Delta Kappan, 73,* 705–708.

U.S. House of Representatives Select Committee on Children, Youth and Families. (1990). *No place to call home: Discarded children in America.* Washington, DC: U.S. Government Printing Office.

Vega, W. A., Kolody, B., Hwang, J., & Noble, A. (1993). Prevalence and magnitude of perinatal substance exposures in California. *The New England Journal of Medicine, 329,* 850–854.

Walker, C. D. (1994). African American children in foster care. In D. J. Besharov (Ed.). *When drug addicts have children: Reorienting child welfare's response* (pp. 145–152). Washington, DC: Child Welfare League of America, Inc.

I

Obstacles to Adoption: The Missing Pieces of the Puzzle

I have witnessed cases in which it appears that the "system"…negotiate[s] a compromise of long-term foster care rather than facing the adversarial issue of termination of parental rights, the leap of faith of legal commitment and the child's own compelling need for legally permanent and lifetime parents. Every child in long-term foster care is vulnerable to growing up without achieving a consistent, lifetime relationship with parents. As such, long-term foster care is a very poor substitute for legal permanency through adoption. [Digre 1994: 11]

To be effective in counseling prospective adoptive parents, professionals need to present current information describing what is known about the effects of prenatal substance exposure on child growth and development, the importance of prevention and intervention, and the nature of substance abuse and addiction. At the same time, professionals need to apply adoption theory and best practice to cases in which prenatal alcohol and/or other drug abuse is a factor. Finally, to help clients make truly informed decisions, professionals must openly acknowledge and present what is not yet known about the extent and impact of prenatal substance exposure. Although this book's primary focus is on informing practitioners about what is known in this complex field, this chapter provides an overview of those areas that remain unclear.

Professionals as well as prospective adoptive parents should be aware that the subject of infants and children with prenatal substance exposure who also may be candidates for adoptive placement is a relatively new area of research and service development. It is equally important to acknowledge that, in the vast majority of cases, available information related to prenatal substance exposure overall does not enable us to predict with certainty the long-term outcome for any individual child. Thus, individuals and families who are considering adopting a child who has been exposed prenatally to alcohol and/or other drugs, along with persons who have already embarked on this road toward building or adding to their families, will all be participants in developing a knowledge base and in helping to create effective service systems for themselves and their children.

There are many more infants and children with prenatal substance exposure whose long-term interests would best be served by adoptive planning than are actually provided with adoption services. Overall, fewer than 10% of children in out-of-home care are adopted, and an even smaller percentage of substance-exposed children find their way into adoptive homes [Quinton et al. 1992]. Yet a significant proportion of children in out-of-home care who do not get placed for adoption also fail to achieve permanency by means of family reunification [U.S. Department of Health and Human Services 1991]. This discrepancy may best be explained by examining the obstacles that block these children's paths to adoption. Out of scrutiny of these roadblocks, it is hoped, strategies for minimizing the obstacles will emerge.

Clarifying the Extent of the Problem

It is unclear how many infants are born with prenatal exposure to alcohol and/or other drugs and are either in adoptive placement or in need of a permanent plan. The vast range among estimates of the number of infants born in this country every year with prenatal substance exposure is in part due to the lack of an empirical national study to determine the incidence of alcohol and other drug use among pregnant women. The figures cited in the introduction to this volume, for example, are based on pilot studies [Feig 1990] or analyses conducted within individual states [Vega et al. 1993]. Moreover, even within the scope of these limited investigations, accurate estimates of prevalence are difficult to obtain because infant symptoms as well as signs of maternal drug use are widely diverse and often missed by medical as well as child welfare practitioners [Feig 1990].

Identification of substance-abusing mothers and infants with prenatal alcohol and/or other drug exposure is challenging on a variety of levels. Substance abusers commonly do not admit their use of drugs due to denial, guilt, and/or fear of consequences. Further, many health care professionals have not had training on addiction or on how to obtain accurate histories from substance-abusing clients. The absence of procedures for routine drug testing in hospitals means that mothers and newborns generally are not tested for alcohol and/or other drug use. Shortened hospital stays following delivery (often as brief as 24 hours) make it difficult for hospital personnel to gather the necessary assessment information about mothers and make detailed observations of their infants. In addition, many substance-abusing women deliver outside of the hospital.

In some cases, women may stop using drugs at some point during pregnancy or shortly before delivery, so that even if urine toxicology testing (the most common form of drug screening) is conducted, it may not yield an accurate picture of the patient's long-term drug history—urine tests can only account for substances used or absorbed within a short period of time before testing [Los Angeles County Department of Health Services, Alcohol & Drug Program Administration 1993; Vega et al. 1993]. More complex and costly methods of drug detection include meconium analysis (testing of the newborn's first stool), which can provide information about maternal substance abuse up to three months prior to delivery [Ostrea et al. 1992, 1993], and maternal hair analysis, which can provide information about substance abuse over varying lengths of time. Because evidence of drug use remains in the hair, longer hair samples provide extensive information on past substance abuse (hair normally grows about one centimeter per month) [Marques et al. 1993]. Stringent laboratory guidelines must be followed, however, to derive accurate information from any of these techniques. In short, the high cost of universal screening of all women at delivery and methodological problems in identifying those women who should be screened [Tronick & Beeghly 1992] make identification of children with prenatal substance exposure difficult.

Information about the number of children with prenatal substance exposure who have been placed in adoptive homes is also not readily available. Many women who use drugs are never identified as being substance abusers and it is frequently difficult to identify infants exposed prenatally to drugs on the basis of their symptoms. Also, statistics keeping is clouded even when mothers have made clear plans to relinquish their newborns for adoption (often through independent adoption). Those involved in the adoption process may inadvertently omit—or may not be sufficiently scrupulous in—history taking and screening for substance exposure, as they do not want to complicate adoption plans. Further contributing to this lack of accurate data is the fact that most child welfare agencies do not keep statistics on this topic.

The ambiguous status of children with prenatal substance exposure within the child welfare system also presents problems in determining the number of substance-affected children who would be candidates for adoptive placement if the obstacles to placement were eliminated. Many agencies and individual practitioners erroneously assume that children with prenatal drug exposure are not adoptable or at least are not adoptable until a long-term prognosis can be established. Thus, they do not effectively and aggressively recruit adoptive homes for them [Child Welfare League of America 1992]. This impediment is compounded by the reality that many children find themselves in legal limbo for extended periods of time because of their biological parents' chronic and long-term problems related to substance abuse. Termination of parental rights in these situations can take as long as three years or more [Jones et al. 1992]. By the time it is even considered, legal guardianship or long-term family foster care in the child's current placement is often pursued instead of adoption because the child may be in a situation from which it would be very painful to separate, or the child may have become deeply troubled as a result of too many moves and/or inconsistent caregiving in the past. Even though in many of these circumstances adoptive placement would have been the most beneficial option, these children cannot be counted in adoption statistics regarding children who were exposed prenatally to drugs.

Finally, it is important to recognize that the child welfare system does not achieve permanency for a great many children who are in need of such a plan, for various reasons: lack of funding, inadequate resources, poor training, and the overwhelming number of children in need of permanency planning. This is especially the case when parental abuse of alcohol and/or other drugs is involved [Child Welfare League of America 1992].

Lack of Certainty Regarding Long-Term Outcomes

In many instances, the first obstacle that presents itself on the road to adoption for infants and children with prenatal substance exposure is ambivalence and uncertainty on the part of professionals regarding future prospects—that is, the adoptability—of these children. This attitude is commonly shared by professionals from an entire range of disciplinary specialties, including social services, the legal system, medicine, nursing, psychology, and child development. Practitioners in all of these fields might prefer to wait for definitive, long-term findings to guide their work, but such conclusive findings are not available to date. It is not unusual, therefore, for infants with prenatal substance exposure to be left in out-of-home care for extended periods of time due to professionals' hopes or expectations that another evaluation at some later point will yield a clear prognosis and detailed information to present to prospective adoptive parents. This occurs repeatedly, despite all we know about the critical importance of stable caregiver-infant attachment during the first year of life [Coyne & Brown 1985], and despite our knowledge that waiting months or even over a year will rarely furnish significantly more helpful or definitive diagnostic or prognostic information on a child than was available at the outset.

The case vignette on the following page illustrates some potential consequences of this ambiguity about planning for children in situations of prenatal substance exposure, especially with respect to the lack of certainty regarding long-term outcomes.

Clearly, this high-risk infant with no parental or extended family involvement would have been best served by active pursuit of adoption during the first year of life, with adoptive parents who were fully prepared, as well as of the same race and culture as the child. The child's placement with the foster mother was fraught with problems and the risk of impermanence: there were no relatives or

Case Vignette

Maria was born with prenatal drug exposure and was released directly from the hospital into the care of a 60-year-old widowed foster mother. This foster mother, who was already caring for several children with developmental delays, was of a different race and culture than Maria, had several health problems, and expressed no interest in adopting this child. Maria's biological mother had three other children, all of whom had also been exposed prenatally to drugs and were in out-of-home care. The biological mother had not made visits to any of her children, and shortly after Maria's birth, lost contact with the agency. Maria's paternity was unclear. Although Maria's foster mother was fond of the child, she told the child welfare worker that she felt the infant should be placed for adoption quickly, both to prevent her [the foster mother] from becoming too attached to the child and to promote the child's best interests. Maria was exhibiting slight developmental delays and some muscle tightness, however, and the juvenile court decided to wait for further developmental evaluation results. Eighteen months later, when Maria was a toddler, the foster mother requested guardianship, and it was granted.

close friends who were willing to assume responsibility for Maria's care in the event that the foster mother became incapacitated; the foster mother felt quite taxed by the needs of all the children in her care and had little time to advocate and attend to each child individually; and the foster mother showed no interest in extending herself to educate Maria about her cultural heritage, or in contacting other individuals who could provide this experience for the child. Finally, the additional time that elapsed while the court awaited a subsequent developmental evaluation only prolonged Maria's stay in care, and lessened the willingness of the foster mother to part with the child. Among other factors, the uncertainty regarding Maria's developmental outcome kept the system from seeking early adoptive planning with an appropriate, prepared candidate.

In addition to children such as Maria, there are many children who were exposed prenatally to alcohol and/or other drugs about whom a great deal of background information is available, whose potential limitations resulting from the prenatal substance exposure may be minimal, but who are kept waiting for homes and denied the permanency of adoptive placement.

Outcomes for Individual Children Are Never Foreordained

Each human being has a unique genetic code that we have as yet no way to predetermine or fix, even when we know that the code entails some risks. We do know, nevertheless, how to enrich our children's lives. We know, for example, that a supportive and responsive family environment is vital in fostering healthy development. We also know that consistency is a critical element in helping children develop trust and a sense of self-efficacy. We know further that community is important in helping children develop a sense of social connectedness and roots. Finally, we know that parents who openly and actively encourage and provide opportunities for growth help their children attain a better quality of life.

Just as we cannot untangle any given child's genetic code, we also are unable to differentiate the complex impact of prenatal substance exposure upon a child's future health and well-being. All investigators basically agree that exposure to alcohol or illegal drugs at any time during pregnancy can be detrimental to the developing fetus in varying degrees [Tyler 1992]. There is general agreement, as well, that a great deal of neurological development takes place after birth [Quinton et al. 1992], and that the outcome for a child with prenatal substance exposure depends largely upon the complex and dynamic interactions between his or her unique biological strengths and vulnerabilities and the influences that are present in his or her social environment—including family characteristics, caregiving, stability, nutrition, intervention, medical care, and cultural factors [Barth 1991; Myers et al. 1992]. Thus, although our inability to predict outcomes for individual newborns who have been exposed prenatally to alcohol and/or other drugs can be frustrating for prospective adoptive parents who want to know as much as possible about the infants they are considering rearing to adulthood, adoptive applicants might in fact be encouraged to know that they can have a very positive impact on the life of a child. Whether the family is of low-, middle-, or upper-income, we know that all children do better when the home environment is nurturing and responsive [Sameroff & Chandler 1975].

Complicating Factors in Assessing the Effects of Prenatal Substance Exposure

Perhaps the primary complication in predicting outcomes for individual children with prenatal substance exposure involves the difficulty of differentiating among the specific effects of various substances of abuse, as polysubstance abuse (use of multiple drugs) is almost universal among substance abusers. Although substance abusers may prefer one drug in particular, they may use other available substances, including alcohol, marijuana, and/or tobacco. In some instances, substance abusers may purposely combine different drugs to achieve a particular effect. The challenge of teasing out the effects of different drugs is monumental [Rodning et al. 1989; Tronick & Beeghly 1992; Tyler 1992]. Adding to this difficulty is the reality that illegal drugs are generally diluted on the streets (for example, cocaine is frequently laced with phencyclidine [PCP] or various "designer" drugs). Most individuals who abuse substances are unaware of both the exact amounts of a given drug they have been taking and of the other substances that may have been mixed into the drug.

In addition, it is almost impossible to determine the timing and frequency of substance use. Not only do substance abusers commonly deny the actual extent of their use, they also frequently lose track of the length of time between doses. Further, binge use may even cause users to forget what they have taken over a period of several days. Current screening methods cannot provide information as to frequency, chronicity, duration, and severity of drug use [Myers et al. 1992; Tronick & Beeghly 1992]. Moreover, any effort to accurately predict the effects of prenatal substance abuse on the developing fetus and the child would have to incorporate information about the timing of use during the mother's pregnancy. Binge use, for example, may have a different impact than sporadic use throughout pregnancy. Likewise, heavy use during the first trimester, when the fetus's organ systems are forming, may have different effects than heavy use during the third trimester, when organ systems are in place and fetal growth is rapidly proceeding.

Other maternal conditions further complicate our ability to predict the effects of substance abuse. Even if it were possible to ascertain precisely which drug(s) the mother took, as well as the dosage, frequency, and timing of use (and this information is almost never available in actual practice), individual differences among pregnant women affect the ways in which various drugs are metabolized. These differences can result in varying degrees of fetal exposure even among women with identical patterns of use [Tronick & Beeghly 1992]. Furthermore, maternal nutritional status, prenatal health care, and exposure to sexually transmitted as well as other communicable diseases (e.g., tuberculosis) also may have a positive or negative impact on how substances affect the unborn child [Corkery 1992; Mayes et al. 1992].

Likewise, individual differences also may alter the ways in which alcohol and other drugs are metabolized by the developing fetus and child. A large number of newborns with prenatal substance exposure, for instance, show no visible symptoms of their condition, while other newborns appear to be clearly impaired. In addition, many of the potential long-term effects of prenatal exposure to alcohol and/or other drugs may not become apparent for years— effects that may include learning problems that only become evident during the school years. To date, no clear correlation has been established between the extent of an infant's withdrawal symptoms and his or her future development. One infant may be extremely irritable and jittery for a few weeks or even for months, and yet later demonstrate normal development; another infant with prenatal substance exposure may exhibit no symptoms initially but may experience significant developmental problems later on. The same lack of correlation between status at birth and future development applies to the results of infants' urine toxicology screens. These screens indicate drug exposure only during the 72 hours prior to testing. An infant with a positive screen for cocaine may later experience few, if any, discernible long-term sequelae; another child who was exposed prenatally to cocaine but who did not have a positive screen may suffer lifelong complications associated with the exposure.

An additional obstacle to determining the long-term effects of prenatal substance exposure on children's development is the insufficient sensitivity of current standardized measures for evaluating infant and toddler development. These instruments cannot identify children who will have mild mental retardation, normal intelligence associated with learning disabilities, or subtle cognitive and behavioral deficits. Although existing measures can determine the presence of a physical disability (such as cerebral palsy), moderate to severe mental retardation, and moderate to severe visual and hearing impairments in very young children, most learning disabilities cannot be detected until the school years [Fried & Watkinson 1990; Taylor & Warren 1984], and few studies have followed children over an extended period of time.

Finally, attempts to study the long-term impact of prenatal substance exposure on children's growth and development are complicated by the difficulty of untangling the effects of intrauterine drug exposure from the effects of other pre- and postnatal influences, including psychosocial, environmental, and hereditary factors. Child development research over the past 20 years has repeatedly confirmed the critical part parenting and the social environment play in contributing to children's developmental outcomes (social, cognitive, and emotional) [Beckwith 1990; Mayes et al. 1992; Tronick & Beeghly 1992]. For example, parental substance abuse is frequently associated with homelessness, violence, child abuse and/or neglect, repeated out-of-home placement of children, and poverty [Bays 1990; Famularo et al. 1992; Mayer & Black 1977; Regan et al. 1987]. Teasing out the effects of these variables from the effects of prenatal alcohol and/or other drug exposure is fraught with complexities.

Methodological Problems Inherent in Substance Abuse Research

Conducting research in the field of addiction is no simple matter. One of the most significant obstacles is the difficulty of obtaining sample populations from which one can generalize to the total population of pregnant women who abuse drugs [Mayes et al. 1992]. Understandably, researchers have used samples that are accessible and convenient, that have a visibly high rate of addiction, and that can be recruited quickly by referral from health care, social service, and protective services agencies [Howard & Beckwith, in press]. Thus, most of the studies that have been conducted to date, aside from those dealing with Fetal Alcohol Syndrome, have focused on low-income women [Myers et al. 1992; Tronick & Beeghly 1992] and women who are chronic and heavy users [Howard & Beckwith, in press]. Few studies have examined women with extensive financial and psychosocial resources, women whose use is primarily "recreational," or women who are just beginning to use drugs [Howard & Beckwith, in press]. Although studies have been conducted with women enrolled in drug treatment programs, for sampling purposes it also is important to study mothers who are not participating in treatment [Deren 1986; Myers et al. 1992].

Moreover, almost no information is available about the impact of paternal substance abuse on the developing fetus, infant, and child. Methodologically, conducting studies on fathers is even more complicated than investigating infants and mothers. At present, researchers have been unable to truly separate out the nature and extent of the substance-abusing biological father's contribution to the outcome for the child.

That widespread cocaine abuse is a relatively recent phenomenon also contributes to research problems. Cocaine became a popular substance of abuse during the mid-1980s, and no prospective studies of the long-term consequences of prenatal cocaine/polysubstance exposure (following children into adolescence) have been published to date [Mayes et al. 1992]. Also, because cocaine is most commonly used in combination with other drugs, definitive information regarding the long-term effects of prenatal cocaine exposure on children's development and growth is lacking [Mayes et al. 1992].

No published reports as yet have described the long-term development of children with prenatal substance exposure who are being reared in adoptive homes. There is also no way of determining whether infants with prenatal substance exposure who are placed for adoption fit into the categories of subjects who have been formally studied to date, or whether they represent another spectrum of the population, where studies may be lacking.

Although some of these methodological problems are complex and technical, they are important to mention here. The lack of definitive findings about the long-term effects of prenatal exposure to alcohol and illicit drugs means that adoptive parents of infants so exposed must be prepared to live with a great deal of uncertainty and ambiguity—a subject discussed in depth elsewhere in this book.

Contradictory Media, Research, and Clinical Reports

The media rarely portray in a realistic balanced way the risks and potentials faced by children exposed prenatally to alcohol and/or other drugs. They have focused even less often on the adoption of children whose biological parents abuse alcohol and/or other drugs. In the professional literature, research findings convey scant information about the adoption of children exposed prenatally to alcohol and/or other drugs. Despite general agreement about the interaction among biological and environmental factors influencing child growth and development, researchers and clinicians disagree among themselves regarding the extent to which protective factors and strengths in the family environment can mitigate the effects of the biological insult associated with prenatal substance exposure. At one end of the continuum are those who contend that the environment, including caregiving, represents the overriding factor. At the other end are those who subscribe to the belief that the biological insult is more significant, long-lasting, and difficult to moderate than environmental influences. Other experts' beliefs lie somewhere between these two views. Because the data available to the general public about these children are confusing at best, it is no wonder that prospective adoptive parents have difficulty learning what is known about the effects of prenatal substance exposure, what is not known, putting it all together in the context of the benefits and challenges involved in building a family through adoption, and making informed and thoughtful decisions.

The Need for Service and Policy Guidelines

Professionals who work daily with the realities of child welfare practice know that the influx into the system of young children who have been affected by their parents' substance abuse and who are in need of permanent homes has had a profound impact on adoption services during recent years. Because work with this population is an emerging field, however, available statistics, professional research findings, reports about intervention strategies, and the incorporation of such knowledge into practice lag far behind the tremendous need. No national statistics exist regarding the number of children with prenatal substance exposure who are currently in adoptive placement. Available statistics reflect only the general category of special-needs adoptions, and prenatal drug exposure represents but one subgroup among special-needs adoptions. Educated guesses and estimates almost certainly fall short, because so many infants with prenatal substance exposure are never identified as such. For children who are identified, obstacles to adoption are so numerous that it is not possible to calculate how many actually would be candidates for adoptive placement if the impediments were diminished or eliminated.

Problems Inherent in Chemical Dependency

Service and policy-related obstacles to the adoption of children with prenatal alcohol and/or other drug exposure frequently have their source in the biological parents' substance abuse problem. In the grip of chemical dependency, many parents find it difficult or even impossible to plan ahead for their unborn or existing children, to provide day-to-day care for their children, to deal with the realities and expectations of the out-of-home care system, or to pursue adoptive placement. Even for parents who are in treatment for chemical dependency and actively struggling with recovery, the goal of achieving abstinence often requires all of their effort and attention, making it difficult for many to care for their children. Although over the past few years increasing emphasis has been placed on preserving and strengthening families, treating chemically dependent parents in a holistic way, and teaching parenting skills as part of a comprehensive substance abuse treatment plan, some parents find undertaking the parental role impossible, too difficult, or not desirable in their foreseeable future. For these individuals, there is seldom sufficient networking, expertise, or even permission within the substance abuse treatment community, the family preservation networks, or the medical profession, to sensitively and knowledgeably explore all avenues toward adoption planning, or to refer the parents to other professionals who could provide expertise. Also, perhaps because so many chemically dependent women suffered deprivations during their own childhoods, their longing to have a traditional family of their own is often very strong and quite hard to abandon, even in the face of mounting evidence that their dreams are not likely to materialize within a time-frame that would be appropriate for their child. Some parents go in and out of multiple treatment programs, appearing only sporadically in the children's lives but not actually abandoning them. Often, they contest termination of parental rights, even in situations where they clearly cannot care for their children and have not been active participants in planning for their children's welfare.

Despite these obstacles, however, many chemically dependent women actually do recognize the extent and severity of their disability and its impact on their ability to parent effectively, and they do relinquish their children voluntarily. Although numbers are not available, clinical experience regarding the sensitivity exhibited by some mothers, despite all of the hardships they must endure, is often quite moving, as the case vignettes on the following pages illustrate.

Agencies and the courts are often reluctant to take the critical and final step of involuntary termination of parental rights when so many chemically dependent parents have not had the benefit of timely access to available, knowledgeable, and effective assessment, intervention, substance abuse treatment, and rehabilitation/relapse prevention programs [Child Welfare League of America 1992]. The paucity of resources for this population of parents and children has caused a significant service gap in meeting their needs.

In addition, the legal time frames for terminating parental rights and providing permanency for children are not always compatible with the problems inherent in drug addiction. This reality creates serious conflicts for individuals who are on the front lines in terms of making decisions in these situations. Chemical dependency is a long-term, chronic condition in which relapses are the rule rather than the exception. Even when substance abusers are sincerely motivated to maintain abstinence and give such efforts their all, they often go through many treatment programs over a long period of time and experience frequent relapses before achieving prolonged abstinence and the ability to parent their children competently. In cases where children are biologically at risk due to prenatal substance exposure as well as emotionally vulnerable due to repeated losses and separations, the biological parents' preparations for resuming parenting responsibilities are further complicated and delayed.

Also, during the lengthy process of rehabilitation, it is difficult to predict which parents will be successful in achieving recovery and

Case Vignette

A substance-abusing mother's two children with prenatal substance exposure were placed in family foster care. The youngest child was three years old. The court mandated that the mother become drug-free in order to regain custody. After many struggles and hardships, including living on the street for periods of time, the mother entered a drug treatment program and stayed clean for four months. Nevertheless, the court terminated her parental rights because of the length of time between the initial order to maintain abstinence and her successful beginning participation in substance abuse treatment. Although extremely sad about this decision, the mother expressed her feelings in a meaningful and clear letter to her children and sensitively participated in a farewell visit.

becoming effective parents and which parents will not. Many involved professionals find it extremely difficult to give up on a biological mother who is making some efforts, because, with enough time, she might be one of those who does make it and resumes care of her children. Unfortunately, many substance-abusing parents do not achieve abstinence, and their children grow up in the deep freeze of limbo, which often means repeated out-of-home care placements, with the accompanying separations, losses, and probable impairments in attachment and trust.

Moreover, even children who do not experience multiple placements may develop a strong attachment to a primary caregiver who may be unable or unwilling to adopt. Thus, a dilemma worthy of Solomon emerges—professionals have to decide whether to sever an attachment and re-place the child in an adoptive home, or whether to leave the child in a placement that does not hold the promise of security and permanency that only adoption can offer. It has been the authors' experience that, because professionals have the added uncertainty regarding long-term outcome in cases of prenatal substance exposure, the balance many times tilts toward long-term out-of-home care or guardianship rather than adoption planning for these children.

Case Vignette

A 30-year-old woman who had been using alcohol and other drugs since she was 14 years old tried to give up drugs during pregnancy but was unable to abstain. The baby's father also had a long-term history of substance abuse. This mother subsequently gave birth to an infant with prenatal drug exposure who was placed in a family foster home directly after hospital discharge. The mother was sensitively offered appropriate and accessible services to help her reunite with her child. Having been raised in foster homes herself, however, the biological mother wanted something different for her child and decided to give up her rights as a parent.

Summary

It is only during the past decade that we have begun to confront the needs of children exposed prenatally to alcohol and/or other drugs and their families in terms of providing services to their caregivers, be they biological families or foster families, and only in recent years has kinship care been formally identified as an important resource for children who cannot be cared for by their biological parents. It is past time for service providers to incorporate this new knowledge and experience into practice in behalf of the growing number of children with prenatal substance exposure whose situations require adoptive placement.

Although missing puzzle pieces, risks, and unknowns are involved in the adoption of infants and children who were exposed prenatally to alcohol and/or other drugs, not to place these children with well-prepared, well-supported, sensitive, and stable adoptive families entails far greater risks to the children, as well as to our society. For every child—but particularly for these children, many of whom are indeed at risk but also have considerable potential—a caring, consistent, and stable environment early on can bring out the best, while the absence of such an environment can, in turn, be detrimental.

References

Barth, R. P. (1991). Trends and issues: Educational implications of prenatally drug-exposed children. *Social Work in Education, 13,* 130–136.

Bays, J. (1990). Substance abuse and child abuse: Impact of addiction on the child. *Pediatric Clinics of North America, 37,* 881–904.

Beckwith, L. (1990). Adaptive and maladaptive parenting: Implications for intervention. In S. Meisels & J. Shonkoff (Eds.), *Handbook of early childhood intervention* (pp. 53–77). New York: Cambridge University Press.

Child Welfare League of America. (1992). *Children at the front: A different view of the war on alcohol and drugs. Final report and recommendations of the CWLA North American Commission on Chemical Dependency and Child Welfare.* Washington, DC: Author.

Corkery, L. (1992). Prenatal exposure to drugs of abuse: What we know and don't know about developmental outcome. *Newsletter of the Clearinghouse for Drug Exposed Children, 3*(1), 3, 5–7.

Coyne, A., & Brown, M. E. (1985). Developmentally disabled children can be adopted. *Child Welfare, 64,* 607–615.

Deren, S. (1986). Children of substance abusers: A review of the literature. *Journal of Substance Abuse Treatment, 3,* 77–94.

Digre, G. P. (1994, May 5). Obtaining permanency/provision of quality care: Ownership of permanency planning decision making. *Special information: Department of Children's Services update.* Los Angeles: Department of Children's Services.

Famularo, R., Kinscherff, R., & Fenton, T. (1992). Parental substance abuse and the nature of child maltreatment. *Child Abuse & Neglect, 16,* 475–483.

Feig, L. (1990, August). *Drug-exposed infants and children: Service needs and policy questions.* Washington, DC: U.S. Department of Health and Human Services, Office of the Assistant Secretary for Planning and Evaluation (unpublished report).

Fried, P. A., & Watkinson, B. (1990). 36- and 48-month neurobehavioral follow-up of children prenatally exposed to marijuana, cigarettes, and alcohol. *Developmental and Behavioral Pediatrics, 11*(2), 49–58.

Howard, J., & Beckwith, L. (in press). Issues in subject recruitment and retention with pregnant and parenting substance-abusing women. In L. Rahdert (Ed.), *Treatment for drug-exposed women and children: Advances in research methodology.* Rockville, MD: National Institute on Drug Abuse (NIDA monograph).

Jones, R. L., McCullough, C., & Dewoody, M. (1992). The child welfare challenge in meeting developmental needs. In S. L. Quinton, S. A. Johnson, E. M. Johnson, R. W. Denniston, & K. L. Augustson (Eds.), *Identifying the needs of drug-affected children: Public policy issues* (pp. 109–132). Rockville, MD: Office for Substance Abuse Prevention; U.S. Department of Health and Human Services (OSAP prevention monograph 11, DHHS publication number (ADM) 92–1814).

Los Angeles County Department of Health Services, Alcohol & Drug Program Administration (1993). *Fact sheet: State of California—Perinatal substance exposure study.* Los Angeles: Author.

Marques, P. R., Tippetts, A. S., & Branch, D. G. (1993). Cocaine in the hair of mother-infant pairs: Quantitative analysis and correlations with urine measures and self-report. *American Journal of Drug and Alcohol Abuse, 19*(2), 159–175.

Mayer, J., & Black, R. (1977). Child abuse and neglect in families with an alcohol or opiate addicted parent. *Child Abuse & Neglect, 1,* 85–98.

Mayes, L. C., Granger, R. H., Bornstein, M. H., & Zuckerman, B. (1992). The problem of prenatal cocaine exposure: A rush to judgment. Commentary. *Journal of the American Medical Association, 267,* 406–408.

Myers, B. J., Olson, H. C., & Kaltenbach, K. (1992). Cocaine-exposed infants: Myths and misunderstandings. *Zero to Three, 13*(1), 1–5.

Ostrea, E. M., Jr., Romero, A., & Yee, H. (1993). Adaptation of the meconium drug test for mass screening. *The Journal of Pediatrics, 122,* 152–154.

Ostrea, E. M., Jr., Brady, M., Gause, S., Raymundo, A. L., & Stevens, M. (1992). Drug screening of newborns by meconium analysis: A large-scale, prospective, epidemiologic study. *Pediatrics, 89,* 107–113.

Quinton, S. L., Johnson, S. A., Johnson, E. M., Denniston, R. W., & Augustson K. L. (Eds.) (1992). Introduction. In *Identifying the needs of drug-affected children: Public policy issues* (pp. 1–10). Rockville, MD: Office for Substance Abuse Prevention; U.S. Department of Health and Human Services (OSAP prevention monograph 11, DHHS publication number (ADM) 92–1814).

Regan, D. O., Ehrlich, S. M., & Finnegan, L. P. (1987). Infants of drug addicts: At risk for child abuse, neglect, and placement in foster care. *Neurotoxicology and Teratology, 9,* 315–319.

Rodning, C., Beckwith, L., & Howard, J. (1989). Characteristics of attachment organization and play organization in prenatally drug-exposed toddlers. *Development and Psychopathology, 1,* 277–289.

Sameroff, A. J., & Chandler, M. J. (1975). Reproductive risk and the continuum of caretaking casualty. In F. D. Horowitz, M. Hetherington, S. Scarr-Salapatek, & G. Siegel (Eds.), *Review of child development research* (vol. 4) (pp. 184–244). Chicago: University of Chicago Press.

Taylor, R. L., & Warren, S. A. (1984). Educational and psychological assessment of children with learning disorders. *The Pediatric Clinics of North America, 31,* 281–296.

Tronick, E. Z., & Beeghly, M. (1992). Effects of prenatal exposure to cocaine on newborn behavior and development: A critical review. In S. L. Quinton, S. A. Johnson, E. M. Johnson, R. W. Denniston, & K. L. Augustson (Eds.), *Identifying the needs of drug-affected children: Public policy issues* (pp. 25–48). Rockville, MD: Office for Substance Abuse Prevention; U.S. Department of Health and Human Services (OSAP prevention monograph 11, DHHS publication number (ADM) 92-1814).

Tyler, R. (1992). Prenatal drug exposure: An overview of associated problems and intervention strategies. *Phi Delta Kappan, 73,* 705–708.

U.S. Department of Health and Human Services, Office of the Inspector General (1991). *Barriers to freeing children for adoption.* Washington, DC: Author.

Vega, W. A., Kolody, B., Hwang, J., & Noble, A. (1993). Prevalence and magnitude of perinatal substance exposures in California. *The New England Journal of Medicine, 329,* 850–854.

II

Health and Developmental
Considerations

In adopting any child, prospective adoptive parents will have questions about the biological mother's pregnancy, the events surrounding the baby's birth, and the immediate postnatal course. Parents need to have this background information: it may have implications for the child's future health and development, and it will be asked for when parents make appointments for routine well-baby and well-child care, as well as when enrolling their children in child day care, preschool, and/or school programs. Additionally, if the child becomes ill at some point, knowing about these early experiences helps adoptive parents provide useful information to the health care team.

This chapter describes the most common health concerns that have been observed in children who were exposed prenatally to alcohol and/or other drugs, presenting information derived to a large extent from a National Center on Child Abuse and Neglect User Manual written by the authors' staff team [Kropenske et al. 1994]. It begins with a discussion of birthweights and their influences on the infant's current and future medical status, since maternal cocaine abuse has been associated with premature labor and delivery as well as with intrauterine growth retardation. Additional health-related topics include the unique behaviors that have been observed among very young infants with prenatal substance exposure; the infectious diseases that commonly present among populations of adults who abuse alcohol and/or other drugs (since these also may have implications for a substance-abusing mother's offspring); the increased risk for Sudden Infant Death Syndrome (SIDS) among infants with prenatal substance exposure; Fetal Alcohol Syndrome (FAS); and medical follow-up recommendations. The discussion of developmental patterns includes an overview of the usual developmental course, as well as information about the emerging patterns of development that have been observed among children with prenatal drug exposure.

Health Concerns

Birthweight

Birthweight is an important factor associated with children's overall health and development. Many studies have found that birthweight can be a potential indicator of acute as well as long-term medical conditions, and also of temporary as well as permanent developmental impairments in groups of children studied to date [Boyle et al. 1993; McCormick et al. 1992; Saigal et al. 1994; Breslau et al. 1990; Gibson et al. 1990a; Gibson et al. 1990b; Hack et al. 1994; Szatmari et al. 1990; Victorian Infant Collaborative Study Group 1991]. Children who are born full-term (that is, after 37 to 42 weeks' gestation) and who weigh over five and one-half pounds (2500 grams) at birth are less likely to have serious medical problems following delivery and are more likely to exhibit normal development as compared to children who are born preterm or small for gestational age (whether preterm or full-term).

Prematurity

Prematurity is defined as birth at less than 37 weeks' gestational age. The majority of preterm infants weigh less than 2500 grams. Although preterm delivery generally occurs in less than 10% of the newborn population, the risk of prematurity among substance-exposed infants is higher [Chasnoff et al. 1987; Zuckerman et al. 1989]. Research over the past 25 years has demonstrated that prematurity in and of itself—without the added risk factor of prenatal substance exposure—poses a distinct set of biological risks that can result in chronic illness for the infant and interfere with normal growth and development [Cohen et al. 1992]. Moreover, the recent development of new medical technology within neonatal intensive care units has promoted the survival of newborns weighing as little as 500 grams (about one pound). Thus, in studying the health and development of these children, researchers are now viewing birthweights among premature infants in terms of their association with medical and developmental outcomes. Findings include the following:

- Low birthweights are associated with an increase in acute medical complications following birth and with extended periods of hospitalization [Boyle et al. 1983].

- Birthweights under three pounds (501 to 1000 grams) have been associated with poor physical growth and poor general health status at school age [McCormick et al. 1992; Saigal et al. 1994].

- Low birthweight infants are at increased risk for neurosensory deficits [Gibson et al. 1990b], behavioral and attention difficulties, psychiatric problems, and resulting poor school performance when they reach school-age [Breslau et al. 1988; Gibson et al. 1990a; Hack et al. 1994; Szatmari et al. 1990; Victorian Infant Collaborative Study Group 1991].

Prospective adoptive parents should understand, however, that even among children born preterm and with low birthweights, a nurturing and responsive caregiving environment and early intervention can mitigate some of these biological risks [Beckwith 1990; Brooks-Gunn et al. 1992].

Aside from low birthweight, acute medical complications associated with preterm birth include intracranial hemorrhages, bronchopulmonary dysplasia (BPD), retinopathy of prematurity (ROP), respiratory distress syndrome (RDS), and disorders that interfere with normal feeding ability. The term "medically fragile" is commonly applied to infants who display some of these conditions. In some cases, however, the illness may be short-lived and the child may outgrow this status. In other cases, largely depending upon the severity of the illness, the child may have long-term health and/or developmental problems.

Intracranial Hemorrhages

Intracranial hemorrhages refer to bleeding into the brain tissue. Not only is this condition more common among children born preterm than those born full term, it also has been reported to occur with increased frequency among infants with cocaine exposure who were born prematurely and with very low birthweights [Singer et al. 1994]. This condition is known to be a risk factor for future physical, sensory (hearing and vision) [Pike et al. 1994], and/or intellectual problems, depending upon the location and severity of the bleed. Cerebral palsy or impaired motor ability, for example, can occur when there has been an intracranial bleed or an interference with the blood flow to areas of the brain that govern movement. If the bleed occurs in areas of the brain governing cognition, there is an increased risk that the child may suffer future cognitive impairments, ranging from very mild to severe.

Hydrocephalus is another complication that may result from an intracranial hemorrhage. It occurs when the hemorrhage obstructs the normal flow of cerebral spinal fluid that circulates around the nervous system and causes serous fluid to accumulate within the cranium. Hydrocephalus can interfere with physical and/or intellectual development. Treatment for hydrocephalus involves the surgical insertion of a ventricular peritoneal (VP) shunt, or tube, which provides drainage of the fluid from the brain into the abdominal cavity. Such a shunt may be required throughout the child's lifetime and requires ongoing follow-up from neurological specialists to ensure that the tube does not become obstructed or infected.

Bronchopulmonary Dysplasia

One of the most well-recognized complications of prematurity is bronchopulmonary dysplasia (BPD), a condition that affects lung tissue and interferes with normal breathing functions. Following their discharge from the neonatal intensive care unit , children with this condition may continue to require oxygen, have complex medication regimens, and need special home-monitoring of their heart and respiratory rates. Children with BPD are at increased risk for poor weight gain, serious respiratory tract infections, multiple hospitalizations, and delayed development [Robertson et al. 1992]. Furthermore, this condition requires that parents learn to use any necessary equipment, administer medications, detect signs of respiratory infection, and be able to administer cardiopulmonary resuscitation in the event that the child experiences periods of apnea (prolonged cessation of breathing).

Retinopathy of Prematurity

Preterm infants are at risk for developing retinopathy of prematurity (ROP), a disease involving the blood vessels in the eye. Although multiple causes of this disorder have been suggested, no specific cause has been identified to date, and no fully adequate treatment modalities have been developed. All preterm infants should receive a thorough eye evaluation by an ophthalmologist before they are discharged from the nursery in order to determine the severity of the condition; they will also need ongoing follow-up eye examinations until the condition has stabilized. In some cases, ROP improves over time and children do not suffer visual impairment. In other cases, however, children may be left with varying degrees of visual handicap and may require early intervention programs to help them learn about their environment through tactile and auditory channels as well as through their remaining visual abilities.

Interferences with Normal Feeding Ability

Several conditions—including low birthweight in the absence of additional medical complications—may interfere with an infant's ability to feed. A baby weighing under three pounds, for example, may require a special soft nipple to obtain an adequate supply of nourishment without fatigue until additional weight is gained. Moreover, the presence of medical complications may further impair an infant's ability to take nutrition by mouth. If an intracranial bleed has resulted in interferences with the movements that coordinate sucking and swallowing, the caregiver may need to consult with an occupational therapist to learn positioning and physical support techniques that will enable the baby to suck and swallow normally. If the interferences are severe, additional medical measures may have to be taken to make sure that the baby has adequate nutrition and weight gain. Infants with BPD may expend too many calories working to breathe or may become short of breath while feeding. In such cases, supplemental gavage/forced feeding (formula given through a small tube that passes through the mouth or nose into the stomach) may be required, and parents will need special training on using this equipment.

Intrauterine Growth Retardation

The term *intrauterine growth retardation* (IUGR) is used interchangeably with *small for gestational age* (SGA) to describe fetuses whose growth is suboptimal for their gestational age (usually, this means that the infant's birthweight is below the third percentile for his or her gestational age—or that 97% of infants at the same age are heavier than the infant) [Harel et al. 1993]. IUGR can occur in full-term as well as in preterm infants, and it is not uncommon for infants who were exposed prenatally to alcohol and/or other drugs to exhibit this condition [Chiriboga 1993]. Causes for IUGR vary. The most common causes are conditions that result in decreased nutrition for the fetus during pregnancy. Maternal hypertension (high blood pressure), for instance, frequently causes constriction of the blood vessels, including those that lead from the placenta to the fetus, thus restricting the transport of nutrients that are important for growth. Such hypertension may be the result of genetic predisposition, obesity, and/or stress, but drugs such as cocaine, methamphetamine, and PCP may also bring about this condition. Insufficient maternal caloric intake may also result in inadequate fetal nutrition and IUGR—it is not uncommon for women who abuse cocaine to experience decreased appetite and thus provide inadequate nutrition for themselves and their unborn children. IUGR may also be associated with congenital infections (that is, infections that are present during pregnancy and passed on to the fetus) such as rubella, cytomegalovirus (CMV), syphilis, or HIV. Extensive research on infants with IUGR who have not been exposed to drugs has shown that:

- Preterm infants who also have IUGR are at even greater risk for future health and developmental problems than preterm infants without IUGR [Martikainen 1992].

- Full-term infants with IUGR are at greater risk for future health and developmental problems than full-term infants whose birthweights are appropriate for their gestational ages [Gazzolo et al. 1994].

Failure To Thrive

Failure to thrive (FTT) is a syndrome of disordered growth and development characterized by a marked deceleration in weight gain and a slowing in the acquisition of developmental milestones [Drotar 1988]. Infants may not gain weight for a variety of reasons. Medical reasons resulting from biological causes may include vomiting, excessive diarrhea, poor swallowing, cystic fibrosis, and congenital heart disease. Infants also will fail to gain weight if they are given insufficient protein and calories, which may occur if the caregiver mixes formula improperly, does not feed frequently enough, or fails to respond to the infant's signals when he or she is hungry. FTT can also result from psychosocial deficits in the caregiver-infant relationship, such as failure to provide adequate physical nurturing in the form of contact comfort (holding, cuddling, or touching).

In infants who were exposed prenatally to alcohol and/or other drugs, FTT may be due to both medical and environmental factors. A pattern of poor sucking, swallowing difficulties, and distractibility has been observed in many of these infants. In addition, children who live in dysfunctional, chemically involved families are at increased risk for parental neglect and for consistently receiving inadequate nutrition. Finally, some infants who were exposed prenatally to drugs are born very small for gestational age and, in spite of adequate caloric intake, may never attain average growth parameters.

Accurate diagnosis of FTT often entails hospitalization to determine its exact causes. In cases of environmental FTT, once adequate calories and/or appropriate nurturing care are provided to the child, rapid weight gain usually occurs. Unfortunately, this simple medical treatment cannot be effective on a long-term basis unless a thorough evaluation is made to determine the reasons for the child's poor weight gain.

In cases of environmental FTT, an individualized, interdisciplinary treatment program should be established to deal with the interrelated needs of both the parent and the child. The program may include any or all of the following: parent education; individual, conjoint, and/or family counseling; medical services; and substance abuse treatment. Close in-home monitoring also can be an important support for the family as well as an essential safeguard when the child remains within the parental home.

Neurobehavioral Symptoms

A variety of unique neurological behaviors have been noted in newborns who were exposed prenatally to alcohol and/or other drugs. The most commonly observed symptoms include irritability, tremors or jitteriness, prolonged or high-pitched crying, increased or decreased muscle tone, alternating periods of lethargy and irritability, frantic sucking of hands, uncoordinated sucking, and disturbances in sleep patterns.

Within 72 hours after birth, the majority of infants who were exposed prenatally to heroin and/or methadone demonstrate withdrawal symptoms of irritability and tremulousness. Although these symptoms often decline over the first month of life, some narcotic-exposed infants remain symptomatic for as long as nine months. Initially, newborns may also have red, dry skin on their knees, elbows, and cheeks as a result of their excessive body movements. In addition to these symptoms, infants who were exposed prenatally to heroin and/or methadone often experience fever, sweating, diarrhea, excessive vomiting, and even seizures [Finnegan & Wapner 1987]. Medication for symptomatic infants is warranted when vomiting or diarrhea results in weight loss or dehydration. These newborns may also require medication to calm them, and to help them suck and swallow more successfully. Most of these symptoms abate by the first three months of life, although others may linger. Among preterm infants with very low birthweights, some of these symptoms may be masked due to muscle weakness and other complications associated with premature birth.

Infants who were exposed prenatally to stimulants, such as cocaine and methamphetamine, show a different pattern of behaviors. They may appear lethargic during the first few days following birth [Mayes et al. 1993]. When such infants are alert, however, they are often easily overstimulated and may progress from sleep to a state of loud crying within seconds. As they become older, infants who were lethargic during the immediate postnatal period often become increasingly irritable and difficult to console. These behaviors, however, tend to decrease over time and often have been observed to subside by late toddlerhood [Dixon et al. 1990].

Infectious Diseases

Infants with prenatal substance exposure may often be exposed either prenatally or at the time of delivery to infectious diseases contracted by their mothers. Mothers who have multiple sexual partners, a history of prostitution, or a history of intravenous drug use are at increased risk of acquiring a variety of infectious diseases that can be passed to their children. Because many of these infectious agents cross the placenta, infants are at increased risk of acquiring their mothers' infections in utero. The most commonly seen infectious diseases in infants of substance abusers, when the substance abusers have had multiple sexual partners, are gonorrhea, syphilis, herpes, chlamydia, hepatitis B, human immunodeficiency virus (HIV) and/or acquired immunodeficiency syndrome (AIDS), and multidrug-resistant tuberculosis (TB). Prospective adoptive parents should find out from the health care team whether a diagnostic evaluation has been undertaken to determine the presence of any of these diseases, what treatment has been given, and what additional treatment will be required.

Sudden Infant Death Syndrome (SIDS)

Children who have been exposed prenatally to alcohol and/or other drugs are at increased risk of dying from sudden infant death syndrome (SIDS) [Kandall et al. 1993]. SIDS (sometimes called "crib death") is defined as the sudden death of an infant under one year of age that remains unexplained after autopsy, investigation of the death scene, and review of the case history [Ariagno & Glotzbach 1991]. In the United States, SIDS is the leading cause of death in infants between one and 12 months of age. SIDS may have multiple causes and its occurrence is almost impossible to predict. Children who die from SIDS commonly exhibit no other sign of illness immediately before their death.

Home apnea/cardiac monitoring is recommended for preterm infants who experience recurrent apnea and for full-term infants who have had "severe acute life-threatening episodes," sometimes referred to as "near-miss SIDS." The decision to institute home monitoring should be based on medical assessment and reached in collaboration with the caregiver. There is no guarantee that SIDS can be prevented, and it can occur in spite of appropriate monitor use. Caregivers of children who require apnea monitors must be able to perform cardiopulmonary resuscitation.

Fetal Alcohol Syndrome (FAS)

Alcohol is commonly abused by pregnant women who abuse illicit drugs. According to one recent study, a large percentage of women whose primary substance of abuse is cocaine report that they also drink to the point of intoxication [Howard et al. 1995].

Alcohol consumption during pregnancy may result in a pattern of birth defects known as Fetal Alcohol Syndrome (FAS) [Hansen et al. 1978; Jones & Smith 1973]. A diagnosis of FAS is based on three factors: prenatal and postnatal growth retardation, including low birthweight and microcephaly (abnormally small head); central nervous system abnormalities, including intellectual impairment, developmental delays, behavior dysfunction, and neurological abnormalities; and abnormalities of the face, including small eyes, short eye openings, epicanthic folds, flat upturned nose, indistinct philtrum (groove in the midline of the upper lip), thin upper lip, crossed eyes, droopy eyelids, and external ear malformation [Smith 1979]. Over the long term, children with FAS have been observed to have significant disabilities, including impaired cognition, learning disorders, and emotional problems [Brown et al. 1991; Streissguth et al. 1990].

Children with a confirmed history of prenatal alcohol exposure, who display some of the symptoms associated with FAS but who do not meet all of the diagnostic criteria, are referred to as having Fetal Alcohol Effect (FAE). Among children with FAS or FAE, it has been suggested that the incidence of anomalies corresponds with the amount of alcohol consumed by the mother during pregnancy [O'Connor et al. 1986; Streissguth et al. 1989]. Furthermore, even among children who have a history of prenatal alcohol exposure but who have normal intelligence and minimal physical abnormalities, problems with learning, attention, memory, and problem-solving are common, and poor coordination, impulsiveness, and hyperactivity have also been reported [Shaywitz et al. 1980].

Careful monitoring of growth as well as screening for any additional physical problems that may accompany either FAS or FAE are required for all affected children so that appropriate services can be provided. Moreover, involvement in an early intervention program for children with special needs is also recommended for children who exhibit developmental delays.

Recommendations for Medical Follow-Up

All newborns who have been exposed prenatally to alcohol or other drugs require careful medical follow-up. Children who were prenatally substance-exposed may develop some of the medical conditions described above. Therefore, they require careful observation. Thus, whenever possible, arrangements should be made for the parent or caregiver to visit the hospital before the infant's discharge to learn about the child's special needs and to receive instruction in any special caregiving requirements. People who are contemplating adopting a child with prenatal drug exposure may find it helpful to clarify the nature and extent of any potential health risks by asking the following questions of the health care team:

- Has the baby suffered any complications (related to prematurity or low birthweight, for instance)?

- Was there a medical evaluation to determine the severity of these complications?

- Is there evidence that the baby is improving and that the conditions are resolving, or is there evidence of potential permanent impairment?

- Does the baby have any special caregiving needs relating to these conditions? If so, what are these needs and what will need to be done to meet them?

- Based upon the health care team's experience with other infants who have had similar conditions, what is the baby's medical course anticipated to be?

Additionally, the adoptive parents should be provided with a written summary of the infant's diagnoses and medical complications after birth, the treatments that were provided, and the follow-up care that will be necessary. This is especially critical for those infants who will not be receiving their medical follow-up from practitioners who are familiar with their histories.

Children who were exposed prenatally to alcohol and/or other drugs should have more frequent pediatric well-baby care than is customary. An initial appointment should be made with the child's pediatrician within two weeks after discharge. Subsequent well-baby appointments should be scheduled at one, two, four, six, eight, ten, and 12 months. This increased frequency is desirable in order to give caregivers extra support and to provide any anticipatory guidance. Frequent medical follow-up also enables close monitoring of the child's ongoing physical care. For infants who are medically fragile, pediatric well-baby care is especially critical. In addition to subspecialty follow-up, such infants also require regular well-baby follow-up with a primary care physician to ensure that appropriate immunizations and preventive health care services are provided.

Developmental Patterns

Infants and children who have been exposed prenatally to alcohol and/or other drugs are at increased risk for developmental problems. These risks have been described in a variety of review publications [Bays 1990; Brooks-Gunn et al. 1994; Deren 1986]. Like the medical conditions described above, some of these developmental patterns may have a limited course, while others may persist over the long term. To date, the majority of preschool-age children with prenatal substance exposure who have been enrolled in research projects have been found to exhibit developmental patterns that fall within the normal range, although some have demonstrated patterns that indicate a potential risk for future learning disabilities. A small percentage of children with prenatal substance exposure have been found to have moderate to severe developmental impairments.

Regardless of their health status, all children with prenatal substance exposure should be evaluated from a developmental standpoint at least once during the first six months of life, again at 12 months, and at least every year thereafter until they reach school age, when their development generally will be monitored by the education system. Developmental follow-up is critical for children with prenatal alcohol and/or other drug exposure because early intervention and early identification of developmental problems are key to optimizing social, language, cognitive, and motor development. As has been demonstrated in other high-risk groups of children (e.g., preterm children, children born small for gestational age, and children with diagnosed physical and/or mental disabilities), infants who experience responsive caregiving environments and young children who are enrolled in center-based programs generally show better developmental outcomes than children who do not have these experiences [Beckwith 1990; Brooks-Gunn et al. 1992; Shonkoff & Meisels 1990]. Through home-, center-, and school-based programs, children who were affected by their biological parents' substance abuse can be exposed to enriched environments and given opportunities that will foster their development.

Developmental Assessment

A variety of specialists—including pediatricians, occupational therapists, and psychologists—use standardized tests such as the Bayley Scales of Infant Development, the Gesell Developmental Schedules, and the Denver Developmental Screening Test to evaluate infants' and young children's personal/social, language, adaptive/cognitive, and motor skills. Such evaluations provide information about children's current strengths and problem areas and may suggest future problems with moderate to severe mental retardation. They are not sufficiently sensitive, however, to identify a particular child who may subsequently exhibit short attention span, learning disability, hyperactivity, or other developmental problems over time.

Beginning when children are about three years old, standardized intelligence quotient (IQ) tests such as the Wechsler or the McCarthy scales are used to evaluate cognitive abilities. Measures such as the Achenbach Child Behavior Checklist are used to assess social and behavioral problems in preschool age and older children. Though these measures help to identify warning signs (e.g., delayed language development, poor fine motor coordination, hyperactivity, short attention span) for future learning difficulties, they indicate *risk status* only and cannot be used to predict specific learning problems. Only during the school-age years can precise measures be used to detect existing learning disabilities (e.g., attention deficit disorder, dyslexia, etc.) in a child.

Developmental Patterns of Prenatally Drug-Exposed Children

Infants and young children with prenatal drug and/or alcohol exposure display a wide range of developmental patterns, varying from normal to deviant. It bears repeating that these patterns are the result of complex interactions among biological and environmental factors. Though we can do little to alter the course of biological events, we can often reduce the impact of biological risks by promoting nurturing, responsive, and healthy caregiving environments.

Infancy (0 to 15 Months)

UNPREDICTABLE SLEEPING PATTERNS: Most infants develop predictable sleeping patterns by four to six months of age. Although newborns generally sleep for short periods of time throughout the 24-hour cycle, infants generally are able to sustain a six- to seven-hour nighttime sleep pattern at some point between four and six months of age. Some infants who have been exposed prenatally to alcohol and/or other drugs continue to demonstrate the sleeping patterns that are considered typical of a newborn throughout the first year.

FEEDING DIFFICULTIES: By the time they are two weeks old, most infants have established a somewhat regular pattern of feeding and are able to suck effectively enough to have regained their birthweight. Infants who were exposed prenatally to alcohol and/or other drugs, however, may experience a variety of feeding difficulties, including a need for prolonged feeding time due to uncoordinated and ineffective sucking movements or lethargy, distractibility during feeding, frequent spitting up of formula, and an increased need to suck (hyperphagia).

IRRITABILITY: Newborns in general exhibit a range of temperaments. Some infants are generally easygoing and can be readily soothed when fussy; others tend to be irritable and hard to calm. Infants with prenatal substance exposure often display such irritability, and caring for these infants may be difficult. Moreover, these infants may be easily overstimulated and, once aroused, may have great difficulty calming themselves.

ATYPICAL SOCIAL INTERACTIONS: Social interactions begin at birth. When awake, newborn infants respond to voices by turning toward and visually connecting with the caregiver. These are brief behaviors, but they are especially rewarding to parents because they begin the attachment process. By four months of age, infants typically coo in response to social exchanges, make direct eye contact, and have a social smile for persons in the immediate environment. At six months of age, the highly social child becomes increasingly discriminating and smiles only infrequently at strangers. In contrast, infants who have been exposed prenatally to alcohol and/or other drugs may exhibit a number of atypical social responses, including indirect gaze, gaze aversion, and less marked stranger discrimination during the second half of the first year of life than is exhibited by nonexposed infants.

DELAYED LANGUAGE DEVELOPMENT: Language development during early infancy involves cooing, smiling, chuckling, squealing, and crying. Infants with prenatal substance exposure, however, may demonstrate fewer vocalizations and less babbling than nonexposed infants.

INCREASED MUSCLE TONE AND POOR FINE-MOTOR DEVELOPMENT: Motor development follows a similar pattern in all healthy infants, although the age at which individual milestones are normally achieved may vary. Young infants who were exposed prenatally to heroin and methadone generally reach gross motor milestones at appropriate ages, though they frequently exhibit increased muscle tone (stiffness). In contrast, young infants exposed to stimulants such as cocaine may have decreased muscle tone and variable motor development, though most also demonstrate attainment of motor milestones at appropriate ages. Infants nine to 15 months old with prenatal substance exposure may experience problems with fine motor coordination, unsteadiness in the movement of extremities, and mild problems with balance.

Toddlerhood (15 to 36 Months)

ATYPICAL SOCIAL INTERACTIONS: Toddlers see themselves as the center of the universe, and the focus of all activities. The pronoun "mine" epitomizes this particular age. Building trust in the social relationship with the caregiver is an important behavior that is learned during the toddler period; such trust largely determines the success of subsequent social interactions. A child who builds a secure attachment with his or her primary caregiver early on will likely have effective social interactions later in life. Toddlers with prenatal alcohol and/or other drug exposure or those who live in unpredictable caregiving environments may demonstrate atypical social behaviors, including overfriendliness, withdrawal, and impulsivity.

DELAYED LANGUAGE DEVELOPMENT: Although toddlers have an expanding vocabulary, they understand more words (receptive language) than they are capable of speaking (expressive language). Toddlers who were exposed prenatally to substances tend to have decreased vocalizations and immature pronunciation of single words.

MINIMAL PLAY STRATEGIES: Play is a central activity that promotes young children's early cognitive development. As children grow, their pretend-play with dolls, baby bottles, cooking utensils, and trucks becomes increasingly elaborate. Toddlers' interactions with toys and other objects within their environment become purposeful and organized, and their activities are sequenced to include a beginning, a middle, and an end (for example, most toddlers will hold a baby doll, feed it, and then put it to bed). In structured testing situations, however, some children with prenatal substance exposure appear less able than those not so exposed to independently organize a meaningful sequence of play with such common toys.

Preschool Years (Three to Five Years)

Preschoolers are more socially independent than toddlers and are beginning to learn to share and take turns. As they grow, their language skills become increasingly sophisticated, and their attention spans are sufficient to allow them to learn within a group setting that provides less individualized attention than they needed as toddlers. Many preschoolers who have suffered prenatal substance exposure, however, show increased activity levels, short attention spans, impulsivity (easy loss of control), mood swings, and problems with moving from one activity to another. Some substance-affected preschoolers also may continue to demonstrate difficulties in the auditory processing of spoken words as well as the visual processing of material presented to them in the form of pictures. Furthermore, some demonstrate sporadic mastery of tasks, in which the skills they demonstrate one day are absent on another day. Concern about the social development of substance-affected preschoolers also has led to ongoing research into the patterns of attachment and social interaction within this high-risk population of children.

School and Teenage Years

Little is known about the long-term biological effects of prenatal exposure to drugs, and longitudinal prospective studies are needed to build a solid base of pertinent knowledge. Children who exhibit language delays, distractibility, and/or problems with fine motor coordination during the preschool period, however, are at increased risk for learning disabilities during their school and teenage years.

Relatively more is known about the cognitive development of school-aged children with FAS—that is, children who were exposed prenatally to alcohol. By the time such children reach elementary school, many demonstrate cognitive skills that fall within the range of mental retardation. Other affected children display attention deficit disorder and learning problems specific to difficulties with visual and auditory processing.

Despite the absence of research data describing the long-term effects of prenatal substance exposure, professionals can provide services in a number of ways for children and adolescents who were exposed prenatally to drugs. Whatever behavioral symptoms children may demonstrate (and whatever their cause) as they pass from preschool into elementary school and beyond, available testing measures become increasingly sensitive in identifying learning strengths as well as problems. A team of teachers, psychologists, speech and language therapists, hearing and vision specialists, nurses, and other professionals can assess difficulties with learning that may be related to short attention span, speech and language problems, impulsivity, difficulties with short-term memory, auditory and visual processing, and so on. Based on such evaluations, school personnel can work with parents to develop effective educational programs to help the child or adolescent compensate for the identified problems.

In terms of primary prevention efforts, professionals and adoptive parents can:

- Advocate for specialized educational services within the school system, tutoring for academic underachievement, and assessment and intervention for neuropsychological problems.

- Explore recreational and work experiences that will give school-age children or adolescents the opportunity to experience success.

- Participate in parent support groups that provide education and guidance for dealing with difficult childhood and adolescent behaviors.

- Participate in individual and family therapy.

Summary

This chapter provides an overview of the common health and developmental concerns associated with prenatal exposure to alcohol and/or other drugs. Very little is known, however, about long-term outcomes for children with prenatal drug exposure as the youngsters progress beyond the preschool years. We do know that children with Fetal Alcohol Syndrome continue to have impaired cognitive development as they progress through childhood and adolescence, but no investigators have studied the effects of prenatal exposure to other drugs over such an extended span of time.

In general, children who have language delays, fine motor problems, and easy distractibility early on are at risk for learning difficulties in the future, regardless of whether these early problems are related to prenatal substance exposure or whether they stem from entirely different causes. Child development, however, is an ongoing process. Just as early intervention has been shown to have a positive impact, comprehensive, coordinated efforts can be helpful at whatever stage they are begun.

This chapter is not intended to be exhaustive but to offer information in response to some of the most basic questions adoptive applicants have about children with prenatal substance exposure. It also provides a foundation from which adoptive parents can begin to formulate informed questions to raise with their children's health care providers and teachers.

References

Ariagno, R. L., & Glotzbach, S. F. (1991). Sudden infant death syndrome. In A. M. Rudolph (Ed.), *Rudolph's Pediatrics* (19th ed.) (pp. 850–858). San Mateo, CA: Appleton & Lange.

Bays, J. (1990). Substance abuse and child abuse: Impact of addiction on the child. *Pediatric Clinics of North America, 37,* 881–904.

Beckwith, L. (1990). Adaptive and maladaptive parenting: Implications for intervention. In S. Meisels & J. Shonkoff (Eds.), *Handbook of early childhood intervention* (pp. 53–77). New York: Cambridge University Press.

Boyle, M. H., Torrance, G. W., Sinclair, J. C., & Horwood, S. P. (1983). Economic evaluation of neonatal intensive care of very low birth weight infants. *The New England Journal of Medicine, 308,* 1330–1337.

Breslau, N., Klein, N., & Allen, L. (1988). Very low birth weight: Behavioral sequelae at nine years of age. *Journal of the American Academy of Child and Adolescent Psychiatry, 27,* 605–612.

Brooks-Gunn, J., Liaw, F., & Klebanov, P. K. (1992). Effects of early intervention on cognitive function of low birth weight preterm infants. *Journal of Pediatrics, 120,* 350–359.

Brooks-Gunn, J., McCarton, C., & Hawley, T. (1994, January). Effects of in-utero drug exposure on children's development. *Archives of Pediatric and Adolescent Medicine, 148,* 33–39.

Brown, R. T., Coles, C. D., Smith, I. E., Platzman, K. A., Silverstein, J., Erickson, S., & Falek, A. (1991). Effects of prenatal alcohol exposure at school age: II. Attention and behavior. *Neurotoxicology and Teratology, 13,* 369–376.

Chasnoff, I. J., Burns, K., & Burns, W. J. (1987). Cocaine use in pregnancy: Perinatal morbidity and mortality. *Neurobehavioral Toxicology and Teratology, 9,* 291–293.

Chiriboga, C. A. (1993). Fetal effects. *Neurologic Clinics, 11,* 707–728.

Cohen, S. E., Parmelee, A. H., Beckwith, L., & Sigman, M. (1992). Biological and social precursors of 12 year competence in children born preterm. In C. Greenbaum & J. Auerbach (Eds.), *Cross national perspectives in children born at risk* (pp. 65–78). Norwood, NJ: Ablex.

Deren, S. (1986). Children of substance abusers: A review of the literature. *Journal of Substance Abuse Treatment, 3,* 77–94.

Dixon, S. D., Bresnahan, K., & Zuckerman, B. (1990, June). Cocaine babies: Meeting the challenge of management. *Contemporary Pediatrics, 7,* 70–92.

Drotar, D. (1988). Failure to thrive. In D. K. Routh (Ed.), *Handbook of pediatric psychology* (pp. 71–107). New York: Guilford Press.

Finnegan, L. P., & Wapner, R. (1987). Narcotic addiction in pregnancy. In J. R. Neibyl (Ed.), *Drug use in pregnancy* (pp. 203–222). Philadelphia: Lea and Febiger.

Gazzolo, E., Scopesi, F. A., Bruschettini, P. L., Marasini, M., Esposito, V., Di Renzo, G. C., & de Toni, E. (1994). Predictors of perinatal outcome in intrauterine growth retardation: A long term study. *Journal of Perinatal Medicine, 22*(1), 71–77.

Gibson, D. L., Sheps, S. B., Uh, S. H., Schechter, M. T., & McCormick, A. Q. (1990a). Retinopathy of prematurity-induced blindness: Birth weight-specific survival and the new epidemic. *Pediatrics, 86,* 405–412.

Gibson, N. A., Fielder, A. R., Trounce, J. Q., & Levene, M. I. (1990b). Ophthalmic findings in infants of very low birthweight. *Developmental Medicine and Child Neurology, 32,* 7–13.

Hack, M., Taylor, G., Klein, N., Eiben, R., Schatschneider, C., & Mercuri-Minich, N. (1994). School-age outcomes in children with birth weights under 750 g. *The New England Journal of Medicine, 331,* 753–759.

Hansen, J. W., Streissguth, A. P., & Smith, D. W. (1978). The effects of moderate alcohol consumption during pregnancy on fetal growth and morphogenesis. *Pediatrics, 92,* 457–460.

Harel, S., Kutai, M., Tomer, A., Tal-Posener, E., Leitner, Y., Fatal, A., Jaffa, A., & Yavin, E. (1993). Intrauterine growth retardation: Diagnosis and neurodevelopmental outcome. In N. J. Anastasiow & S. Harel (Eds.), *At-risk infants: Interventions, families, and research* (pp. 145–159). Baltimore: Paul H. Brookes Publishing.

Howard, J., Beckwith, L., Espinosa, M., & Tyler, R. (1995). Development of infants born to cocaine-abusing women: Biologic/maternal influences. *Neurotoxicology and Teratology, 17*(4), 403–411.

Jones, K. L., & Smith, D. W. (1973). Recognition of the fetal alcohol syndrome in early infancy. *Lancet, 2,* 999–1001.

Kandall, S. R., Gaines, J., Habel, L., Davidson, G., & Jessop, D. (1993). Relationship of maternal substance abuse to subsequent sudden infant death syndrome in offspring. *The Journal of Pediatrics, 123*(1), 120–126.

Kropenske, V., & Howard, J., with Breitenbach, C., Dembo, R., Edelstein, S. B., McTaggart, K., Moore, A., Sorensen, M. B., & Weisz, V. (1994). *Protecting children in substance-abusing families.* Washington, DC: U.S. Department of Health and Human Services/National Center on Child Abuse and Neglect (user manual series).

Martikainen, M. A. (1992). Effects of intrauterine growth retardation and its subtypes on the development of the preterm infant. *Early Human Development, 28*(1), 7–17.

Mayes, L. C., Granger, R. H., Frank, M. A., Schottenfeld, R., & Bornstein, M. H. (1993). Neurobehavioral profiles of neonates exposed to cocaine prenatally. *Pediatrics, 91*, 778–783.

McCormick, M. C., Brooks-Gunn, J., Workman-Daniels, K., Turner, J., & Peckham, G. J. (1992). The health and developmental status of very low birth-weight children at school age. *The Journal of the American Medical Association, 267*, 2204–2208.

O'Connor, M. J., Brill, N. J., & Sigman, M. (1986). Alcohol use in primiparous women older than 30 years of age: Relation to infant development. *Pediatrics, 78*, 444–450.

Pike, M. G., Holmstrom, G., de Vries, L. S., Pennock, J. M., Drew, K. J., Sonksen, P. M., & Dubowitz, L. M. S. (1994). Patterns of visual impairment associated with lesions of the preterm infant brain. *Developmental Medicine and Child Neurology, 36*, 849–862.

Robertson, C. M. T., Etches, P. C., Goldson, E., & Kyle, J. M. (1992). Eight-year school performance, neurodevelopmental, and growth outcome of neonates with bronchopulmonary dysplasia: A comparative study. *Pediatrics, 89*, 365–372.

Saigal, S., Rosenbaum, P., Stoskopf, B., Hoult, L., Furlong, W., Feeny, D., Burrows, E., & Torrance, G. (1994). Comprehensive assessment of the health status of extremely low birth weight children at eight years of age: Comparison with a reference group. *The Journal of Pediatrics, 125*, 411–417.

Shaywitz, S. E., Cohen, D. J., & Shaywitz, B. A. (1980). Behavior and learning difficulties in children of normal intelligence born to alcoholic mothers. *The Journal of Pediatrics, 96*, 978–982.

Shonkoff, J. P., & Meisels S. J. (1990). Early childhood intervention: The evolution of a concept. In S. Meisels & J. Shonkoff (Eds.), *Handbook of early childhood intervention* (pp. 3–32). New York: Cambridge University Press.

Singer, L. T., Yamashita, T. S., Hawkins, S., Cairns, D., Baley, J., & Kliegman, R. (1994). Increased incidence of intraventricular hemorrhage and developmental delay in cocaine-exposed, very low birth weight infants. *The Journal of Pediatrics, 124*, 765–771.

Smith, D. W. (1979, October). The fetal alcohol syndrome. *Hospital Practice*, 121–128.

Streissguth, A. P., Barr, H. M., & Sampson, P. D. (1990). Moderate prenatal alcohol exposure: Effects on child IQ and learning problems at age 7 1/2 years. *Alcoholism: Clinical and Experimental Research, 14*, 662–669.

Streissguth, A. P., Sampson, P. D., & Barr, H. M. (1989). Neurobehavioral dose-response effects of prenatal alcohol exposure in humans from infancy to adulthood. *Annals of the New York Academy of Sciences, 562,* 145–158.

Szatmari, P., Saigal, S., Rosenbaum, P., Campbell, D., & King, S. (1990). Psychiatric disorders at five years among children with birthweights < 1000g: A regional perspective. *Developmental Medicine and Child Neurology, 32,* 954–962.

Victorian Infant Collaborative Study Group [Kitchen, W., Campbell, N., Carse, E., Charlton, M., Doyle, L., Drew, J., Ford, G., Gore, J., Kelly, E., McDougall, P., Rickards, A., Watkins, A., & Yu, V.] (1991). Eight-year outcome in infants with birth weight of 500 to 999 grams: Continuing regional study of 1979 and 1980 births. *The Journal of Pediatrics, 118,* 761–767.

Zuckerman, B., Frank, D. A., Hingson, R., Amaro, H., Levenson, S.M., Kayne, H., Parker, S., Vinci, R., Aboagye, K., Fried, L., Cabral, H., Timperi, R., & Bauchner, H. (1989). Effects of maternal marijuana and cocaine use on fetal growth. *The New England Journal of Medicine, 320,* 762–768.

III

Origins, Loss, Uncertainty, and Open Adoption: The Client's Perspective

It would appear that adoptive parents need to be more mature and psychologically aware than biological parents because of the special obstacles they face. They need to know more about themselves and to be capable of empathizing with their child's position. [Severson 1991: 96]

All prospective adoptive parents must engage in serious reflection about their own attitudes and beliefs related to adoption, both before making the decision to adopt and during the adoption process. Through this type of reflection, which can be facilitated by careful preparation under the guidance of informed professionals and by participation in support groups, prospective adoptive parents can arrive at a decision that is comfortable for them—whether their decision is to proceed with the adoption, to reflect further, or to put their plans on hold.

One key consideration is the prospective adoptive parents' feelings about the biological parents of the child whom they might be adopting. Another consideration concerns the losses inherent in the adoption process—the prospective adoptive parents' own losses as well as those experienced by the child and his or her biological family. Again, any adoption involves a degree of uncertainty regarding the future, and it is important for prospective adoptive parents to examine their ability to live with these ambiguities. Finally, the option of open adoption and its many variants and nuances must be carefully weighed.

All of these considerations are important in any adoption. For prospective adoptive parents who are contemplating adopting a child who has been exposed prenatally to alcohol and/or other drugs, however, this process of reflection may take on a slightly different focus. It is this focus that is the fabric of this chapter. Professionals who are counseling prospective adoptive parents about the adoption of children with prenatal substance exposure have to be aware of the unique concerns surrounding that exposure if they are to guide their clients productively through the critical self-examination process.

Feelings About Substance-Abusing Biological Parents

Adoptive parents—some with joy and some with anguish—are awaking to the fact that roots, however twisted, are as vital to the leafing of the tree, as is the gentle nurturing of sun and rain. [Severson 1991: 101]

Children's biological origins constitute a significant part of their personal identities [Katz 1980; Kirk 1984]. The key to a child's development of a positive self-image is the ability of the adoptive parents to have and convey to the child an empathic attitude toward their biological parents and relatives. Adoptive parents must be able to empathize with the biological parents' struggles as well as to welcome and be responsive to the searching and sometimes painful questions about their backgrounds that adopted children are likely to raise throughout the various developmental stages. An ease of communication between adoptive parents and adopted children regarding the children's biological parents and the children's early awareness that they have been adopted are among the factors that correlate with adoptees' subsequent healthy adjustment as adults [Kirk 1984, 1985; Weeks et al. 1976].

Nonetheless, most adoptive parents find it difficult and even threatening to talk about adoption with their children; they experience particular anxiety in discussing specifics regarding biological parents. Adoptive parents often find it painful to explain their own infertility or to acknowledge that the child is not biologically their own, possibly due to worries that the child will favor the biological parents above themselves because of blood ties [Schechter 1970]. In other situations, adoptive parents may feel conflicting emotions or even severely disapprove of the circumstances surrounding the child's birth, as their own values and/or conduct in the areas of sexuality and reproduction may be vastly different from those of the biological parents [Kirk 1984; Schechter 1970]. Even when unintended, adoptive parents' negative feelings about biological parents reach their children not only through words, but also through attitudes and behaviors. Thus, consciously or unconsciously, adoptive parents over time may communicate to their children a view of their roots and beginnings as being shameful and humiliating. If the adoptive parents' feelings about the biological parents are accepting, however, they may convey to the children a meaningful and understandable view of their roots [Katz 1980].

Prospective adoptive parents must therefore have opportunities to honestly explore, clarify, and work through their feelings about the biological parents of children who are placed for adoption. Before making a decision to adopt a child with prenatal substance exposure, prospective adoptive parents must express and confront their own attitudes in general about biological parents who abuse alcohol and/or other drugs, and in particular, about women who abuse alcohol and/or other drugs during pregnancy. Prospective adoptive parents must also explore the attitudes and feelings of their extended family members, friends, and social supports regarding chemically dependent parents and children who have been exposed prenatally to drugs. However subtly, these views may influence the parents own attitudes and responses, and also may be communicated—verbally or nonverbally—to the adopted child. So often, professionals who are counseling prospective adoptive parents focus primarily on projected long-term outcomes for children who were exposed prenatally to drugs, failing to attend equally to the ways in which the biological parents are viewed by the adoptive applicants.

Experiences Related to Substance Abuse

Substance abuse, especially abuse of alcohol and/or other drugs during pregnancy, is an intensely emotional and conflict-laden subject for much of the general population, and certainly for prospective adoptive parents. In exploring their experiences concerning alcohol and/or other drug abuse—within both their own personal and cultural backgrounds as well as those of family members and friends—individuals who are contemplating adopting a child with prenatal substance exposure must understand that the actual experiences may not be as significant as the way in which they have been felt, viewed, and reviewed. The way in which adoptive parents have internalized such experiences is likely to influence the way in which they deal with the biological parents' use of drugs. For example, many prospective adoptive parents at one time may have had, or may currently have, a friend or close family member with a substance abuse problem. If such parents have honestly and openly faced their feelings of grief and frustration regarding this serious life experience, their pain may be transformed into a source of strength and self-awareness that can help build empathy with both the adopted child and the biological parents. Kirk [1984] describes this process of developing sensitivity and empathy in relation to some adoptive parents' self-examinations and interpretations of their problems with infertility:

> [R]ecall of one's pain previously suffered can become a vehicle for apprehending the pain in others and their needs for help. Once self-defeating, the pain has become the raw material for the apparatus needed by the adoptive parents who wish to be 'on call' for their child. [p. 159]

Similar processes may occur in situations involving substance abuse.

Adoptive applicants should also explore their own work-related experiences with substance abuse. Individuals who are considering adopting—including those who are also actively struggling with their own childlessness—may find it difficult to work in settings where they have frequent contact with infants and children who have been profoundly affected by their parents' use of alcohol and/or other drugs. For example, physicians and nurses who work in neonatal intensive care units, child protective services workers, police officers, and teachers all may experience intensely painful feelings, including anger and jealousy, in relation to the clients they serve. These individuals may believe strongly in their own potential to be good parents, if only they could conceive, while they daily encounter substance-abusing mothers who readily bear one child after another yet not only are unable to care for their children but also have created lifelong medical and developmental problems for their offspring. Whether the feelings that prospective adoptive parents hold toward biological parents in these kinds of situations are empathic and compassionate, whether they are angry and punitive, or whether they are some combination thereof will be determined by the way in which their own backgrounds and experiences have been incorporated into their attitudes, feelings, and beliefs about substance-abusing biological parents.

Attitudes about Substance Abuse

It is recognized that many people view substance abuse as a moral failure, and some believe that addiction and its related behaviors represent willful misconduct and criminal activity [Child Welfare League of America 1992]. Some individuals believe that substance abuse warrants punitive action, and/or that this problem exists primarily among poor, minority populations [Quinton et al. 1992]. Many persons feel especially angry toward women who abuse drugs during pregnancy because they "knowingly" may be causing irreversible harm to an innocent newborn.

Due to their lack of understanding about the nature and characteristics of chemical dependency, however, persons who hold such negative views may not be able to fathom the power that addiction asserts over every aspect of the substance abuser's life and the central role that addiction assumes. Because of their primary attachment to their substance(s) of abuse, users may engage in prostitution, theft, or other illegal and dangerous behaviors in their quest for drugs. Unplanned pregnancies are common occurrences resulting from such activities; some women may not even be certain about their children's paternity. Many adoptive applicants find it difficult to fully acknowledge and empathize with such a life-style; this is also the case for many substance-abusing parents, who often may be hardest on themselves. For prospective adoptive parents whose own personal deprivations remain unexamined and unresolved, or whose standards of morality, religious beliefs, or other core principles stand in serious conflict with the circumstances of a child's conception and birth, acceptance of the vital importance of such a child's beginnings may not be possible.

Many adoptive parents who believe that substance abuse is a moral failure involving willful misconduct believe that their negative views are directed to the biological parents' behaviors alone. Over time, however, these attitudes also exert a pervasive negative influence on the adopted child. If a child exhibits behavioral problems as he or she grows, for instance, adoptive parents who hold negative views of the parents may attribute these problems to "damaged goods" or "bad blood" originating from the youngster's immoral, impulsive, and promiscuous biological parents [Sorosky et al. 1978]. If adoptive parents consider a child's biological parents to be immoral and weak-willed, they may correspondingly view the child's behavioral difficulties as predictive of other serious behaviors and may overreact with excessive punishment. Unfortunately, the punishment may serve only to further impair the child's already fragile sense of self-esteem. If, instead, adoptive parents are able to remain open-minded to the possibility that the child's behaviors might stem from other causes—for example, physiological overload—they might seek out guidance in modifying the environment and helping the child to develop successful coping strategies [Healey 1993]. The case vignette on the facing page illustrates how this can occur.

Prospective adoptive parents who harbor punitive attitudes toward substance abusers may encounter further difficulties as their adopted child matures. Some adoptive parents may be consumed by overriding fears that a child's potential for addiction will emerge during adolescence. Parents who have unexamined concerns about a child's potential for chemical dependency may express these fears in ways that actually effect a self-fulfilling prophecy—a child may be "driven" into a pattern of compulsive acting-out by the adoptive parents' constant identification of the child with his or her biological parents' problems [Sorosky et al. 1978]. In fact, it is not at all unusual—and it may even be realistic—for parents today to worry about children getting involved with drugs. Certainly, this can be an important concern if there is a family history of substance abuse. In preadoption counseling, therefore, individuals should have the opportunity to explore their attitudes about these aspects of substance abuse as they determine if they will be capable of helping a child deal with related issues over time.

Case Vignette

A five-year-old adopted child had been told repeatedly by his adoptive father that he had to stay within the boundaries of the back yard or else he would be grounded, but the boy kept going beyond those limits. The father thought the child was being defiant and discussed this with the adoptive mother, who, in turn, observed the child playing in the yard. Based on her observation, the mother concluded that the behavior was not an act of defiance, but rather a result of the child's inability to understand the verbal directions. She took the boy's hand and walked him over to the borders of the yard on each side of the house, gently pointing out the boundaries he was not supposed to cross. After this, the child no longer disobeyed. He needed not only to hear the verbal command, but also to be shown in order to process the meaning of this communication.

However thorough this self-examination process may be, not all feelings or their depth can be explored. Living through the years—especially the adolescent years—with adopted children who were exposed prenatally to alcohol and/or other drugs will tap adoptive parents' feelings deeply, prompting them to revisit questions again and again. Sound preparation today, however, lays a foundation for future self-realization, enabling adoptive parents to develop effective approaches for promoting their children's strengths, protective capacities, and self-esteem, while at the same time further educating them and their children about substance abuse prevention in a sensitive and constructive way.

Developing Empathy for Substance-Abusing Biological Parents

If an adopted child does develop problems, whatever their cause, the adoptive parents' anger and frustration can present serious difficulties if their feelings are not tempered by an understanding of the pain and struggles faced by the child's biological parents. In many instances, adoptive parents may ruminate on what the child "might have been" had she or he not experienced such a difficult beginning as in-utero substance exposure, or they may dwell on how much easier and more rewarding it could have been for themselves as adoptive parents if the child had not suffered this adverse intrauterine exposure. In *The Broken Cord*, a factual account of a man who adopted a little boy subsequently diagnosed as having Fetal Alcohol Syndrome, Michael Dorris, the adoptive father and author, describes the pain, frustration, and challenges he experienced in coming to terms with adopting a child who had so many special needs [Dorris 1989]. In chapter after chapter, Dorris writes eloquently about his feelings about the child's biological mother, as well as about women in general who abuse drugs during pregnancy. His feelings of deprivation, sorrow, and anger about the biological mother are commingled with understanding and empathy, which translates into empathy and compassion for the child.

Because an empathic attitude toward parents who are chemically dependent can have such positive significance for the way in which adoptive parents relate to their children, essential questions to explore include the following:

- Do the adoptive parents perceive the biological parents as persons who have their own unique strengths and vulnerabilities in addition to the problem of addiction, or do they stereotype the biological parents simply as "drug addicts"?

- Do the adoptive parents view human behavior as a continuum? Are they aware of their own imperfections and weaknesses, or do they see the substance-abusing biological parents as dehumanized and immoral and thus completely different from themselves?

Adoptive parents should be helped to understand that addiction is a complex problem about which we still know relatively little. The causes of addiction, effective treatment approaches, and the various factors that influence individuals' use and abuse of harmful substances are just not clearly understood. As one recent report noted: "It is the worst of plagues. It knows no season and no boundaries. No mosquito will be identified, no microbe isolated, no vaccine invented to end its reign" [Robert Wood Johnson Foundation 1992: 2]. This knowledge can be humbling, and awareness of these uncertainties can help a person to be nonjudgmental about the overwhelming "pull" and the chronic relapsing nature of addiction, and to focus instead on ways of strengthening protective and compensating factors in the child and his or her environment.

Individuals who hold rigid views of substance abuse as a moral disgrace may find it difficult to conceive of or acknowledge the possibility that a substance abuse problem could arise within their own biological families—in someone as closely related as a sibling or a parent, for example, or even in themselves. Adoptive parents must be made aware that no one is immune to becoming an addict, that given exposure to particular circumstances (such as extreme loss, pain, or stress) and the right substance of abuse, almost any one of us would be capable of developing a chemical dependency. An empathic attitude acknowledges the reality that a vast number of substance-abusing parents themselves have histories that were fraught with family violence, mental health problems, child abuse, parental addiction, economic and emotional deprivation, and major losses. An understanding of how substance abuse so often afflicts those individuals who are already the most vulnerable can lead compassionate individuals to assume the attitude that "there but for the grace of fortuitous and more fortunate circumstances go they" [Kirk 1984: 119].

Patterns of Dealing with Loss

My child was born today,
While another woman felt the wonder of her birth
My heart longed to see her face...
Her family broken, mine begins.
Oh, who can understand the ways of life
When loss and love join hands? [McGuire 1983: 39]

A related and extremely important area for prospective adoptive parents to explore is the various ways in which they have dealt with difficult and/or painful situations and feelings in the past, for these are key in determining whether and/or how they will be able to cope with the range of special needs of an adopted child who has been exposed prenatally to alcohol and/or other drugs.

Loss as an Element of Every Adoption

Loss is at the core of the adoption experience for all parties involved. For prospective adoptive parents, loss and frustration may have occurred—and may still be continuing—in several domains. Some individuals, for example, decide to pursue adoption because of infertility, repeated miscarriages, or genetic/hereditary problems in their family backgrounds. They may harbor concerns about body intactness and/or sexual performance. For most people, these kinds of motivations and situations generally are accompanied by feelings of shame, guilt, alienation, helplessness, and/or anger. The grief they feel—and that they must work through—is most often for the biological child they had originally hoped would be born to them, "a child who carries both one's own genes and one's dreams" [Brinich 1990: 46]. Grief is also a motivating factor for persons who may have decided to adopt because they want to "replace" a child who died, because their other children have grown, because they want more children than they are able to have biologically, because they want a child of a particular gender or a child as a sibling for a biological child, or because they are trying to restore or correct something they feel they missed during their own childhoods. All of these situations involve loss.

Likewise, prospective adoptive parents of children with prenatal substance exposure also must come to terms with their feelings about not adopting the healthy, risk-free baby they might well have preferred. They may need to spend considerable time exploring their feelings about the child's background—with respect to the biological parents' alcohol and/or other drug abuse and related life-style—in terms of the reality of what it is, as opposed to what they might have wanted it to be. In this reflection, they may well again experience a sense of loss.

Personalizing Losses

When adoptive parents personalize the multiple losses associated with adoption, they may feel guilty about having done something "wrong" that has brought about what they perceive to be a punishment (that is, for not having had a biological child, for instance, and for having to take on the extra preparation, tasks, and stresses inherent in adoptive parenthood). Compounding their feelings of deprivation, some prospective adoptive parents may experience resentment and embarrassment at having to demonstrate their suitability to be parents by going through the adoptive application and screening process, as no such demands accompany biological parenthood [Sorosky et al. 1978]. Moreover, adoptive parents are unlikely to experience the traditional supports and ceremonies that usually accompany the birth of a child, nor do they generally receive the same approval, acceptance, and sensitivity on the part of relatives, friends, professionals, and the broader community that are accorded to biological parents [Kirk 1984].

Parents who personalize these losses and continue to feel deprived or defective sometimes want their children to succeed in order to feel adequate and successful themselves. They may perceive a high-risk child who does exhibit special needs as proof of their own inadequacy. One can readily see how serious problems could result if such individuals were to adopt an infant with prenatal substance exposure who did experience difficulties—the adoptive parents may well find themselves unable to provide the support, encouragement, and guidance the child needs in order to maximize his or her own potential.

Transcending Loss

Only by examining their losses and by facing their feelings about frustrated hopes and expectations can prospective adoptive parents in time work through their pain, loss of self-esteem, and anger. As this occurs, they learn not to personalize their losses, but to draw strength from them instead. As Kirk so eloquently describes this process, the pain that previously so consumed adoptive parents "in its new state...will be decontaminated, shorn of its nagging quality" [Kirk 1984: 159]. The pain is not discarded, but rather used to help the adoptive parents understand and acknowledge, both intellectually and emotionally, the differences between biological parenthood and adoptive parenthood.

As feelings of pain lose their negative strength, adoptive parents can use them in a positive way to keep communication open with their children about the realities of being a member of an adoptive family. These parents are better able to see the similarities in all that they, their children, and the biological parents are facing, and to relate with compassion and empathy rather than with denial, anger, and rejection. The greater the empathy the adoptive parents feel toward the child and his or her particular situation, the more compassionate and nonjudgmental their communication with the child about the biological parents will be. As this occurs, parents are likely to feel more satisfied with the adoption, and the child is less likely to feel isolated or to feel that avenues of communication with his or her adoptive parents are closed [Kirk 1984]. Adoptive parents who have faced and worked through their feelings about loss, deprivation, and substance abuse are in a strengthened position to help their children realistically and constructively face their own special losses and experiences related to their biological parents' chemical dependency, their prenatal substance exposure, and the challenges they may be experiencing related to that exposure and to their adoptive status.

Living with Uncertainty

When you decide to have a child, you are hostage to an uncertain future. The fine print of the contract is invisible—it appears, as if inscribed in lemon juice, only under the heat of the bright light of unfolding experience. Control is a delusion, and the only absolutes are retrospective. [Dorris 1989: 198-199]

Just as there are no guarantees for biological parents regarding the future physical, developmental, and psychological health of their children, there are no guarantees for adoptive parents. In fact, for many of the reasons already discussed above, adoption itself puts a child and his or her adoptive parents at increased risk to a certain degree [Katz 1980], even if the biological parents' physical and mental health and the prenatal environment have been quite favorable. In situations involving adoption of infants with prenatal drug exposure, however, even those professionals and researchers who emphasize above all the critical impact of the environment and caregiving practices on the child's outcome agree that prenatal exposure to alcohol and/or other drugs is detrimental and should be avoided if at all possible. Persons who are considering adopting children with prenatal drug exposure must be prepared for and able to tolerate the unique uncertainties and ambiguities that are inherent in such adoptions.

Balancing Optimism with Awareness

To be sure, it is possible that the child will experience no discernible or significant long-term sequelae of prenatal substance exposure, and it can be helpful if parents are optimistic and hopeful that this will be the case. Parents should not look for symptoms of problems everywhere or anticipate problems that might not even emerge, as this kind of overconcern, worry, and vigilance has its own negative impact on the child-parent relationship. Neither is it advisable, however, for parents to go into this type of adoption without being fully aware that children with prenatal drug exposure may be at extra risk; they must be willing, able, and prepared to confront and assume these risks in the event that problems do materialize. Every difficulty that might conceivably arise, how one will feel and react in response, and all the twists, turns, vicissitudes, and challenges that life may present cannot be anticipated. If adoptive parents are aware of the risks involved and of how important it is to be able to live with uncertainties and ambiguities, however, they may feel empowered to examine their own strengths and vulnerabilities and to make informed decisions that they will be able to live with and build upon over time.

Maintaining Objectivity about Media Reports

The difficulty of living with ambiguity and uncertainty and of discerning the strengths and needs of individual children becomes readily evident in media portrayals of children exposed prenatally to alcohol and/or other drugs. Although adoptive parents must be open and receptive to assistance and to suggestions for preventive and remedial interventions if indicated, they also must resist the sway and hysteria of the lay media regarding outcomes and the future of these children. Newspapers and magazines have depicted children with prenatal substance exposure as being hopelessly and irreversibly damaged—as children who were so profoundly affected that they probably would never function in a normal manner in our society. Terms, labels, headlines, and sound bites such as "crack babies," "walking time bombs," or "oblivious to any affection" have been featured prominently. In essence, these pejorative portrayals of the children dismiss them as being without hope, and in effect, discourage many potential caregivers from taking on responsibility for them.

Hearing such language, one can forget that drug exposure is a *risk factor*, not a diagnosis or a specific handicap. When labels such as "drug baby" or "crack baby" are used, the substance exposure is stressed first, and the child comes second. The child's individuality is overlooked. If adoptive parents latch onto such labels and accounts, they may inappropriately lower their expectations of children, or they may attribute any learning or behavioral problems predominately to heredity and prenatal events, even when this may not be the case. By overemphasizing the children's problems as stemming from prenatal exposure to alcohol and/or other drugs, adoptive parents, professionals, and society as a whole may not really examine the influences of other factors—culture, environment, supports, caregiving, and so forth—on the child.

Conversely, several recent articles have asserted that environmental factors can mitigate all or most deficits caused by prenatal drug exposure, and that previous accounts regarding the children's potential deficits and outcomes have been grossly exaggerated. For example, one Los Angeles newspaper featured the headline, "Studies: Drug Babies Doing OK" [Weaver 1994]; another headline stated, "New Research Finds Little Lasting Harm for 'Crack' Children" [Viadero 1992]. It can be equally problematic for adoptive parents of children with prenatal substance exposure to espouse this type of global, one-sided view. One of the risks of not being fully cognizant of the challenges that may lie ahead is that adoptive parents might not provide early intervention to offset problem areas for their children. The adoptive parents' denial of potential risks may even prevent them from identifying problems that early intervention and/or treatment could help. If and when such problems become impossible to deny, parents may feel cheated and overwhelmed, and will lack the benefit of anticipatory guidance that might have been provided had they been more receptive.

Finally, adoptive parents should also be aware of how they perceive the responses of others to media reports. Because of the stigma often attached to substance abuse, the lack of sensitivity and acceptance on the part of others that is so often experienced by adoptive parents overall may be exaggerated when parents adopt an infant with prenatal alcohol or other drug exposure. In other instances, persons who believe reports claiming that children with prenatal substance exposure are at no risk of experiencing adverse effects related to maternal alcohol and/or other drug use may attribute problems to the adoptive parents. As Weiss [1989: 14] has written about parents of children with disabilities of various kinds, "The hurt and pain of seeing our children struggle is intensified when we are blamed and condemned as the cause. It is a double assault. When we need help and support, we often receive just the opposite.... Not only do others blame us, we blame ourselves."

Coming to Terms with Uncertainty

In summary, adoptive parents must not be overly sensitive or responsive to media accounts regarding outcomes for prenatally substance-exposed children, or to the labels that are so often inappropriately attached to these youngsters. Parents moving into this type of adoption must also maintain an attitude of realistic optimism, hoping that the child will be spared serious consequences but accepting the probability that preventive and/or remedial interventions may be necessary and that professional guidance also may be required at times. Such an attitude is quite different from one holding either that the children are "doomed" or that they are "just fine."

Open Adoption

Openness, like many other decisions in parenthood, should be a choice guided and supported by fact and reason. [Berry 1994: 34]

In adopting any child, prospective adoptive parents should consider seriously the risks and benefits of engaging in an open adoption. This section explores the possible advantages and disadvantages of openness in adopting a child who has been exposed prenatally to alcohol and/or other drugs. Two important facts should be kept in mind. First, every situation is unique. Second, it is impossible to anticipate every consequence.

Open adoption has perhaps been most clearly defined by two of its best-known pioneers and advocates, Baran and Pannor, as:

> a process in which the birth parents and the adoptive parents meet and exchange identifying information. The birthparents relinquish legal and basic child rearing to the adoptive parents. Both sets of parents retain the right to continuing contact and access to knowledge on behalf of the child. Within this definition, there is room for greater and

lesser degrees of contact between the parties. The frequency and meaning of the communication will vary during different times in the lives of the individuals involved, depending on their needs and desires and the quality of the established relationship. [Baran & Pannor 1990: 318]

Empirical analysis has been scant, particularly longitudinal research evaluating the impact of the practice of open adoption in general and on children [Baran & Pannor 1990; Barth 1994; Berry 1993b]; studies of open adoption in which the biological parents have abused alcohol and/or other drugs have been even fewer. The usefulness of what little is known is further compromised by the uniqueness of every situation, despite the commonality of chemical dependency. What can be taken under consideration, however, are some of what are believed to be the components of, and requirements for, a successful open adoption; these components can then be integrated with the special considerations faced by all parties to the adoption when the biological parents are chemically dependent and the child has been exposed prenatally to drugs. Reviewing these components provides a framework for exploring the potential advantages and risks of open adoption for each member of the adoption triangle.

Components of Successful Open Adoption

Siegel's [1993] empirical investigation of adoptive parents' perceptions of the initial effects of open adoption on themselves and their infants found that successful open adoptions require trust, honesty, and empathy between the biological parents and the adoptive parents, as well as the ability and commitment on the part of every involved party to put the child's needs before all else and to identify one's own needs and feelings. Another ingredient of successful open adoption is the ability of the biological and adoptive parents to solve problems in mature, responsible, and creative ways.

A further point for consideration in any open adoption is the capacity of all involved individuals to weigh the short- and long-term consequences of initiating and maintaining ongoing contact. Adolescent biological parents, for example, may not be developmentally ready to fully evaluate and anticipate the long-term impact of such openness, focusing instead on the short-term benefits alone. It is often difficult for teenagers to think through the long-term consequences of their behavior and focus on long-term goals [Berry 1993b; Smith et al. 1985].

A survey of a large number of adoptive parents in California whose children were placed with them during the period from 1988 to 1989 [Berry 1993a, 1993b] found that information sharing before placement and contact following placement were fairly common practices, with continued contact most likely to occur with infant adoptions, adoptions where no child maltreatment was known to have taken place, and adoptions by relatives. The researchers also found three important predictors of comfort with openness: (1) the adoptive parents felt they had control over the contacts and had planned and prepared for contact from the beginning of the placement, (2) the adoptive parents had talked with the biological parents before the placement, and (3) the children had no history of maltreatment or prenatal substance exposure. (This third predictor may have been related to the adoptive parents' somewhat negative impressions of abusive or substance-abusing biological parents.) Among adoptions of children with a history of maltreatment or prenatal substance exposure and in which postplacement contacts with biological parents did take place, however, a meeting between the biological and adoptive parents prior to placement was connected with added comfort in postplacement contacts, as compared with adoptions where no such meeting occurred [Berry 1993a, 1993b].

Contraindications for Open Adoption

Kinship Care: A Natural Bridge, a report of the Child Welfare League of America [1994], states that open adoption is probably contraindicated in situations involving serious mental illness, patterns of violence, or extensive substance abuse. The report suggests that such problems within the biological family may be too serious to enable the affected parents to negotiate successfully an open adoption agreement and to fulfill the agreements and responsibilities that are inherent in such adoptions. This would be the case most especially for a full open adoption, in which the biological and adoptive parents meet and share identifying information with each other. In such adoptions, all concerned individuals must consider and decide upon clear expectations, visiting schedules, boundaries, and responsibilities [Sorich & Siebert 1982]. Moreover, these decisions should be

set forth in a written contract, even if such a contract is only morally—not legally—binding.

Parental Substance Abuse and Open Adoption

Prospective adoptive parents of a child with prenatal substance
exposure should reflect on how the considerations and conditions
described above might play themselves out when the biological
parents are chemically dependent. Much, of course, will depend
upon the biological parents' drug(s) of choice, stage of chemical
dependency, and treatment status. It is important to bear in mind,
however, that these factors can vary greatly over the years, as well as
over the short term, and may be difficult to predict. Despite the
commonality of substance abuse, it cannot be overemphasized that
every biological parent and every situation is unique. "Chemical
dependency in the biological family is not necessarily a barrier to
open adoption" [Child Welfare League of America 1992: 162].

Individuals who abuse alcohol and/or other drugs are usually
well aware of the social stigma that so often surrounds their substance abuse, especially during pregnancy, and they often blame
themselves for their illness. Strong feelings of shame, guilt, and low
self-esteem can increase the likelihood that a substance abuser will
minimize the extent of his or her problem or even deny its existence
altogether. Thus, many women who have a substance abuse problem
withhold information about the nature and extent of their drug use,
as well as about their life-styles. Mothers who abuse drugs may also
have fears about criminal or civil actions on behalf of their unborn or
older children [Edelstein & Kropenske 1992; Finkelstein 1990; Jones
1991]; if they are considering adoption for their children, they may
fear that revealing their problem or its true dimensions may prevent
them from obtaining the kind of family and home environment they
want to ensure for their children. Denial and the reasons for it may be
so strong for a pregnant woman who is chemically dependent that
they may interfere with the honesty and trust that are so important
to an open adoption, both in terms of establishing the initial agreement and in carrying it through over the years.

If a woman uses alcohol or other drugs at any time during
pregnancy, her baby is considered to be prenatally drug exposed. Yet
women generally do not set out to harm their babies—in fact, just the

opposite is most often the case. Women who are casual users, women who can stop without great difficulty, or even, in many instances, women who can stop only with considerable struggle, frequently do stop once they find out that they are pregnant. Accordingly, women who continue to abuse substances throughout pregnancy frequently are those who are in an advanced stage of chemical dependency. In such instances, the need for alcohol and/or other drugs is central to the user, and everything else tends to revolve around this priority. Such individuals generally have learned to deal with pain and unpleasantness by taking substances into their bodies to bring about a change in mental status [Kropenske et al. 1994]. In this mental state, it becomes exceedingly difficult for the user to identify feelings and needs, and empathy with others is not readily grasped. For the alcoholic or addict, life often becomes chaotic, unstructured, and unpredictable. Responsible preparation, problem-solving, and follow-through—important elements for an open adoption—are not to be expected from an individual who is chemically dependent to that degree.

Due to chronic and heavy substance abuse and, in many cases, severely deprived and painful backgrounds, biological parents who abuse drugs may have limited or arrested emotional and social development. Many substance abusers report that they began using drugs in early adolescence or even sooner, and their emotional development may not have progressed far beyond that point because they have not struggled and worked through the important stages and tasks associated with adolescence and beyond. If this is the case for a biological parent, then the elements essential to a successful open adoption may be lacking.

Another important consideration is the significant percentage of chemically dependent individuals who suffer from underlying psychiatric disorders that require mental health attention. For many users, substance abuse is an attempt to self-medicate such underlying conditions. It is also possible that a disorder may be the result of long-term addiction and organic damage, or that it may be related to drug or alcohol withdrawal. Even professionals can find it difficult to distinguish among medical conditions, psychiatric disorders, and alcohol and/or other drug abuse problems [Bays 1990; Edelstein & Kropenske 1992; Jessup 1992; Kropenske et al. 1994], although doing so is critical if assessment and treatment are to be effective. To proceed with an open adoption when a biological parent has an undiagnosed and/or untreated psychiatric problem can be risky for all involved.

Violence in a biological parent's background and/or current life situation is another possibility that prospective adoptive parents should explore when considering open adoption. In general, violence is an all-too-frequent occurrence in situations involving substance abuse because of the loosening of controls that individuals experience while under the influence, because of side effects of certain drugs, or because of organic brain damage and/or other medical and physical factors that may be caused or exacerbated by long-term serious substance abuse [Bays 1990; Famularo et al. 1992]. The all-encompassing quest for drugs often involves criminal activities [Bays 1990] that may culminate in violence, even when such actions are not the user's intention. In addition, as noted above, many individuals who abuse alcohol and/or other drugs have experienced physical abuse, neglect, and/or sexual abuse during their childhood and adolescence. As adults, such individuals may become involved in nonnurturing, abusive relationships themselves, and domestic violence may be common.

Because substance abuse tends to be a lifelong problem and relapses are to be expected, it may be difficult for affected biological parents to fulfill ongoing responsibilities toward their children and comply with agreed-upon contracts, no matter how well-meant their intentions. Adoptive parents, in turn, may have difficulty understanding the biological parents' struggles, continuing substance abuse, and related problems with follow-through. In the authors' experience, for example, an adoptive mother and father were distressed and uncertain about how to respond when a biological parent repeatedly asked them for money after visiting with the children. Although the biological parent said that she needed the money for transportation, the adoptive parents feared she might use it to purchase drugs. In other cases, adoptive parents may be concerned that the biological parents' problems will have a negative impact on the children. If ongoing contact is agreed upon as part of the open adoption arrangement, for example, adoptive parents may be concerned that, if contact takes place during the biological parent's periods of sobriety and recovery but is interrupted during periods of relapse, it may cause confusion and feelings of loss for the child [Berry 1993b]. Some adoptive parents may find these issues too problematic and/or painful to deal with and explain, both to themselves and to their children. Other adoptive parents, though, may feel that the risks are worthwhile and that, over time, ongoing contact—even if sporadic—will provide an opportunity for the children to appreciate some of the biological parents' strengths and to understand that the biological parents care, as well as to understand why the biological parents were unable to be effective parents.

In contemplating the pros and cons of open adoption, adoptive parents again may need to reflect upon how they feel and think about maternal substance abuse during pregnancy, especially if the adopted child does have impairments that may be attributed to such exposure. Will ongoing contact with the biological parents help them understand the situation and develop empathy, will it serve to increase their feelings about prenatal substance exposure as a form of abuse, or will it result in some combination of both? Who will there be to help make sense of the inevitably complex and conflicting reactions that will be felt by all involved? The importance of ongoing support is highlighted in the case vignette on the next page.

The potential benefits of open adoption in situations involving chemical dependency include all of the advantages commonly cited for each member of the triad in any adoption, as well as some advantages unique to situations involving parental substance abuse. For biological parents who abuse alcohol and/or other drugs, many of whom have experienced a great deal of loss, pain, and guilt in their lives, an adoption involving some degree of openness may help them assume more responsibility for the arrangement, cope better with the decision to relinquish, deal more effectively with feelings of grief than would occur with a closed adoption, and also relieve some feelings of secrecy, uncertainty, and guilt [Baran & Pannor 1990]. In both the short and the long run, dealing openly, responsibly, and constructively with the adoption may represent an adaptive step in a parent's recovery. For biological parents who have exaggerated fears about the effects of their substance abuse on the child, openness may ease these worries. If the adoptive family is indeed nurturing and stable, the biological parents may also be able to take pride in the

Case Vignette

The foster mother of an 18-month-old toddler with prenatal substance exposure expressed interest in adopting the child, should he become legally free. Meanwhile, the biological mother, who was still using drugs, was permitted weekly monitored visits with her son. Whenever she failed to show up for these scheduled visits, as often happened, the foster mother, intending to be helpful, took the child to visit his biological mother in her apartment to give this mother every opportunity to connect with her child. It took a great deal of counseling and guidance to help this foster mother understand that it was necessary for the biological mother to keep these appointments on her own, that she had to be clean and sober when she visited her son, and that the foster mother, by trying harder than the biological mother, was in fact helping neither the biological mother nor the child.

fact that their decision helped to secure this improved environment for their offspring.

Open adoption can benefit adoptive parents of children with prenatal substance exposure by putting an end to stereotypes about parents who are chemically dependent, instead instilling the acknowledgment that substance abusers are whole and complex people, vulnerabilities and all. In turn, this awareness may help adoptive parents effectively communicate this reality to their children.

For children, an open adoption can potentially dispel some of their ghosts and fantasies about their biological parents, as well as provide valuable information and promote a sense of continuity. Openness can confirm for children that their biological parents did and do care, even if they were or are impaired due to substance abuse, thus reassuring the children that it was the biological parents' problem, not something about the children themselves, that necessitated the relinquishment. Finally, the children can have an opportunity to experience, learn about, and take pride in positive aspects of their biological family background.

As Berry [1993b: 134] noted about open adoption in general, "Given the present state of knowledge, decision-making around open adoption remains a risky business, with substantial need for caution, assessment and planning." What is very clear is that skilled agency/professional services—including but not limited to assessment of the unique aspects of each situation, counseling, support, and mediation—are essential to all of the involved parties during the preplacement phase as well as over the long term following placement. It should also be remembered that there are varying degrees of openness, ranging from the sharing of pictures and developmental information to a fully open adoption [Sorich & Siebert 1982], and that any and all of these alternatives can be explored to suit the best interests of the individual children, adoptive parents, and biological parents involved. Finally, there is a tremendous need for further research on the impact of open adoption in general, and specifically as it relates to the growing number of children whose biological parents abuse alcohol and/or other drugs.

Summary

The considerations brought forth in this chapter are likely to be heavily laden with emotion for prospective adoptive parents. Professionals in preadoption counseling should not only provide opportunities for adoptive applicants to explore their feelings, attitudes, and abilities, but should also assure them that there are no right or wrong responses. Even very supportive and communicative couples may find that each partner brings to the table varying degrees of concern and anxiety; these differences have to be examined in any effort to attempt a resolution.

By helping prospective adoptive parents to clarify their attitudes and expectations, practitioners can guide adoptive applicants toward a successful evaluation of the risks and possibilities involved in adopting a child who has been exposed prenatally to alcohol and/or other drugs. Whether the applicants decide to proceed with the adoption, engage in further reflection, or decline, as long as their decision is reached on the basis of honest and informed consideration they will be assured that they have made the choice that is best.

References

Baran, A., & Pannor, R. (1990). Open adoption. In D. M. Brodzinsky & M. D. Schechter (Eds.), *The psychology of adoption* (2nd ed.) (pp. 316–331). New York: Oxford University Press.

Barth, R. P. (1994). Adoption research: Building blocks for the next decade. *Child Welfare, 73*, 625–638.

Bays, J. (1990). Substance abuse and child abuse: Impact of addiction on the child. *Pediatric Clinics of North America, 37*, 881–904.

Berry, M. (1993a). Adoptive parents' perceptions of, and comfort with, open adoption. *Child Welfare, 72*, 231–253.

Berry, M. (1993b). Risks and benefits of open adoption. *The Future of Children: Adoption, 3*(1), 125–138.

Berry, M. (1994). Parent access after adoption: Should parents who give up their children for adoption continue to have access to them? Yes. In M. A. Mason & E. Gambrill (Eds.), *Debating children's lives* (pp. 20–25). Thousand Oaks, CA: Sage Publications, Inc.

Brinich, P. M. (1990). Adoption from the inside out: A psychoanalytic perspective. In D. M. Brodzinsky & M. D. Schechter (Eds.), *The psychology of adoption* (2nd ed.) (pp. 42–61). New York: Oxford University Press.

Child Welfare League of America. (1992). *Children at the front: A different view of the war on alcohol and drugs. Final report of the CWLA North American Commission on Chemical Dependency and Child Welfare.* Washington, DC: Author.

Child Welfare League of America. (1994). *Kinship care: A natural bridge.* Washington, DC: Author.

Dorris, M. (1989). *The broken cord.* New York: Harper Collins Publishers.

Edelstein, S. B., & Kropenske, V. (1992). Assessment and psychosocial issues for drug-dependent women. In M. Jessup (Ed.), *Drug dependency in pregnancy: Managing withdrawal* (pp. 13–36). North Highlands, CA: California Department of Health Services, Maternal and Child Health Branch (State of California, Department of General Services, Publication Section).

Famularo, R., Kinscherff, R., & Fenton, T. (1992). Parental substance abuse and the nature of maltreatment. *Child Abuse and Neglect, 16*, 475–483.

Finkelstein, N. (1990). *Treatment issues: Women and substance abuse.* Unpublished report funded by the Office of Substance Abuse Prevention (available from the National Coalition on Alcohol and Drug Dependent Women and their Children, 349 Broadway, Cambridge, MA 02139).

Healey, T. (1993). Intervention strategies in children prenatally exposed to drugs...a continuum birth through school age. *The Clearinghouse for Drug Exposed Children Newsletter, 4*(3), 1–3, 6.

Howard, J., Beckwith, L., Rodning, C., & Kropenske, V. (1989). The development of young children of substance-abusing parents: Insights from seven years of intervention and research. *Zero to Three, 9*(5), 8–12.

Jessup, M. (1992). Introduction. In M. Jessup (Ed.), *Drug dependency in pregnancy: Managing withdrawal* (pp. 1–12). North Highlands, CA: California Department of Health Services, Maternal and Child Health Branch (State of California, Department of General Services, Publication Section).

Jones, B. W. (1991). *In-home services: Substance-abusing parents and their children.* Paper presented at the conference on protecting the children of heavy drug users sponsored by the American Enterprise Institute for Public Policy Research, Williamsburg, VA, July 18–21.

Katz, L. (1980). Adoption counseling as a preventive mental health specialty. *Child Welfare, 59*, 161–167.

Kirk, H. D. (1984). *Shared fate: A theory and method of adoptive relationships* (2nd ed.). Port Angeles, WA: Ben-Simon Publications.

Kirk, H. D. (1985). *Adoptive kinship: A modern institution in need of reform.* Port Angeles, WA: Ben-Simon Publications.

Kropenske, V., & Howard, J., with Breitenbach, C., Dembo, R., Edelstein, S. B., McTaggart, K., Moore, A., Sorensen, M. B., & Weisz, V. (1994). *Protecting children in substance-abusing families.* Washington, DC: U.S. Department of Health and Human Services/National Center on Child Abuse and Neglect (user manual series).

McGuire, A. (1983). My child was born today. In P. I. Johnston (Ed.), *Perspectives on a grafted tree: Thoughts for those touched by adoption* (p. 39). Indianapolis, IN: Perspectives Press.

Quinton, S. L., Johnson, S. A., Johnson, E. M., Denniston, R. W., & Augustson K. L. (Eds.) (1992). Introduction. In *Identifying the needs of drug-affected children: Public policy issues* (pp. 1–10). Rockville, MD: Office for Substance Abuse Prevention; U.S. Department of Health and Human Services (OSAP prevention monograph 11, DHHS publication number (ADM) 92-1814).

Robert Wood Johnson Foundation. (1992). *Substance abuse.* Annual report. Princeton, NJ: Robert Wood Johnson Foundation.

Schechter, M. D. (1970). About adoptive parents. In E. J. Anthony & T. Benedek (Eds.), *Parenthood: Its psychology and psychopathology.* Boston: Little, Brown.

Severson, R. W. (1991). *Adoption: Charms and rituals for healing*. Dallas, TX: House of Tomorrow Productions.

Siegel, D. H. (1993). Open adoption of infants: Adoptive parents' perceptions of advantages and disadvantages. *Social Work, 38*, 15–21.

Silverstein, D., & Kaplan, S. (1989). Seven core issues in adoption: A therapeutic framework. In L. Coleman, K. Tibor, H. Hornby, & C. Boggis (Eds.), *Working with older adoptees*. Tustin, CA: Parenting Resources.

Smith, P. B., Weinman, M., Johnson, T. B., Wait, R. B., & Mumford, D. M. (1985). A curriculum for adolescent mothers: An evaluation. *Journal of Adolescent Health Care, 6*, 216–219.

Sorich, C. J., & Siebert, R. (1982). Toward humanizing adoption. *Child Welfare, 61*, 207–216.

Sorosky, A. D., Baran, A., & Pannor, R. (1978). *The adoption triangle*. Garden City, NY: Anchor Press/Doubleday. (Anchor Books Edition 1984).

Viadero, D. (1992, January 29). New research finds little lasting harm for "crack" children. *Education Week, 11*, pp. 1, 10.

Weaver, N. (1994, August 28). Studies: Drug babies doing OK. *Daily News*, p. 12 (serving the San Fernando and neighboring valleys, Woodland Hills, CA).

Weeks, R. B., Derdeyn, A. P., Ransom, J. W., & Boll, T. J. (1976). *A study of adults who were adopted as children*. Paper presented at the annual meeting of the American Association of Psychiatric Services for Children, San Francisco, CA.

Weiss, E. (1989). *Mothers talk about learning disabilities: Personal feelings, practical advice*. New York: Prentice Hall Press.

IV

A Risk and Protective Factors Model

Prospective adoptive parents of children exposed prenatally to drugs must be able to approach the adoption from a viewpoint that stresses strengths, risks, and protective factors, not from a perspective that stresses deficiencies. This means not only recognizing the various risks that are involved, but also emphasizing positives and fortifying elements in the children's backgrounds and current life situations, as well as in the children themselves [Myers et al. 1992]. Embracing this approach requires an ability to individualize each child's strengths and vulnerabilities, advocate assertively for services in behalf of the child to optimize his or her potential, and promote the child's self-knowledge and sense of self-esteem/self-efficacy.

The Child's Experience of Adoption

On some level of his being...[the adopted child] will always feel himself ancestrally abandoned, cosmically alone. [Severson 1991: 4]

The experience of loss is as central to adopted children as it is to biological and prospective adoptive parents. Unlike situations involving divorce or the death of a parent, loss for adopted children is pervasive because adoption usually entails the loss of both biological parents, the extended biological family, and the individual's genealogical and cultural history [Brodzinsky 1990].

People often try to deal with loss by attempting to figure out what they did to cause it; they feel responsible for the loss and try to gain control of future losses. Rather than feeling powerless, children who have been adopted generally personalize the fact of their adoption and view it as a rejection. They commonly feel that they were placed for adoption because they were in some way defective, believing that if they had somehow been better, their biological parents would have wanted them and would not have given them up for adoption [Brodzinsky 1990; Silverstein & Kaplan 1989]. Because of their minority status among the general population, adopted children frequently feel that they are different from other children, and many even feel embarrassed [Sorosky et al. 1978]. They often feel alone with their pain, alienated, incomplete, and disconnected. Feelings such as these can have a damaging effect on children's and adolescents' self-esteem [Brodzinsky 1990].

This sense of being different, incomplete, or defective is exacerbated if conditions and questions related to prenatal substance exposure are not handled sensitively by all parties involved, particularly the child's adoptive parents. The knowledge of having been exposed prenatally to alcohol and/or other drugs produces for the child yet another area about which to feel different, vulnerable, and "not good enough." Family members and professionals who repeatedly use the label "drug baby" in referring to the child, or who attribute age-appropriate difficult behaviors to prenatal exposure to alcohol and/or other drugs, add to the child's self-deprecation about not being the perfect child he or she imagined the adoptive parents would have preferred. For children who actually do have deficits related to prenatal substance exposure, parents' and professionals' exaggerated concerns and fears about these vulnerabilities can promote low self-esteem and a defeatist attitude in the child. For these children, it is important for families and professionals to honestly acknowledge behaviors that indeed are difficult, while at the same time provide encouragement and help in solving problems that arise.

Adopted children in general are susceptible to identity problems and confusion because they have experienced a break in continuity with their past [Silverstein & Kaplan 1989; Sorosky et al. 1978]. These problems can be exacerbated when, as often happens, the children are not given complete information about their biological families. Information gaps may result from actual unknowns about the family history, from adoptive parents' anxiety and discomfort about the biological parents' backgrounds, or from agencies' reluctance to pass on complete and comprehensive information. Secrecy and lack of communication, however, can interfere with the development of a coherent sense of self in adopted children, allowing distortions and inaccurate perceptions to be perpetuated, finally making it difficult for such children to resolve their losses [Brodzinsky 1990].

In situations involving substance-abusing biological parents and the life-styles so often associated with alcoholism/addiction, adoptive parents and professionals must respond knowledgeably and with empathy to help children assimilate information about their backgrounds in a positive way and not to promote feelings of guilt and shame about their birth circumstances. This is particularly important in cases where painful information must be conveyed— for instance, information about a parent's incarceration, or about a parent's illness or death due to overdose, HIV infection, or violence. Again, judgmental, withholding, or punitive attitudes on the part of adoptive parents can breed discomfort, fear, and avoidance in the adopted child.

Uncertainty about the capacity of relationships to be enduring is a related matter that commonly causes anxiety among adopted children in general. Because they may be afraid of experiencing yet another loss, adopted children may be much more vulnerable to feelings of separation, rejection, and abandonment than children who were not adopted [Silverstein & Kaplan 1989]. Adopted children may worry that because they were given up by their biological parents, they may be given up again, this time by their adoptive families [Sorosky et al. 1978]. Such feelings can be intensified for children with prenatal substance exposure who are experiencing difficulties and who sense the frustration of those around them. All children take in far more than adults often realize, as shown in the case examples on the following pages.

Case Vignette

A six-year-old adopted child accidentally overheard her adoptive mother talking about her sibling having been exposed prenatally to drugs, and about some potential problems that caused the mother concern. Afterward, the child asked if she, too, would have problems, since both children had the same biological mother. While acknowledging the biological mother's drug use, this adoptive mother reassured the child by praising her daughter's successful school performance and positive relationships with friends, and by expressing confidence that these achievements would continue.

Maintaining a Balanced View

It is our unspoken messages that our children carry into their future. Our faith becomes theirs; our humor shows them the brighter side. [Weiss 1989: 139]

As noted in many contexts throughout this book, it is vital for adoptive parents to remember that every child with prenatal substance exposure is unique and that one must be realistic yet optimistic about each child's individual potential. Adoptive parents need to seek out and value their children's own special strengths, and then provide experiences through which the children can achieve success at each developmental level. In doing this, parents must maintain a delicate balance between conveying hope and confidence that a child can progress, on the one hand, and not overly pressuring the child about achievement, on the other hand. Similarly, parents must be both patient and persevering if a child is experiencing learning problems, developmental delays, or difficulty making transitions—all of which are commonly observed problems among children who were exposed prenatally to alcohol and/or other drugs. On the basis of several studies, it is clear that a more significant number of children with prenatal substance exposure will require special education services and/or other assistance of a therapeutic nature, such as speech therapy than will children in the general population [Fink 1992; Howard et al. 1989; Young et al. 1992].

Case Vignette

Another child with prenatal drug exposure, who had been placed for adoption at an early age, underwent a disrupted adoption because the adoptive parents were not prepared or equipped to handle the child's needs. When this occurred, the child was returned to the foster parents who had cared for him during the first few months of his life. Although this foster family has since adopted him, during the first year after he returned to their home the child engaged in a great deal of acting-out behavior to test whether these parents would give him up just as his biological parents, then these foster parents, and then his first adoptive parents had done. Over and over again, these very sensitive and committed foster/adoptive parents had to reassure the child that this would not happen again, no matter how much he acted out.

Research has also shown that, in general, many adoptive parents have high, even perfectionist, expectations of their children, and that these may be particularly rigid with respect to academic achievement [Sorosky et al. 1984]. Adoptive parents of infants with prenatal substance exposure must be willing to accept small gains, and be prepared to adjust both short- and long-term goals for the child. Flexibility and the ability to modify expectations—always advisable in parenting—are among the most necessary characteristics for adoptive parents with this population of children.

A delicate balance is also called for between flexibility in terms of social and academic expectations for the child and the necessity of providing the child with structure, clear expectations, and consistent behavioral consequences. Although these qualities may seem contradictory, they are actually complementary. Parents have to be able to modify their goals and expectations in order to fully realize and celebrate their child's actual potential and strengths, instead of basing their goals and expectations on what they wish these strengths were. When adoptive parents are able to express pleasure in their children's actual strengths, the children are able to incorporate these positive responses into their own feelings of self-esteem/self-efficacy. How children feel about their strengths and vulnerabilities is as important—if not more so—than what these strengths and vulnerabilities actually are [Miller 1994].

Advocating for Services

Perhaps drug-exposed children are categorically different than other children who have been adopted before them. Many are neither clearly handicapped nor normal....Knowing that a child has Down syndrome or spina bifida is accompanied by a far clearer view of the child's life course than is knowledge that a child has perinatal drug-exposure. [Barth 1991: 326]

Children with prenatal substance exposure often fall between the cracks of existing service delivery systems for various reasons. First, as Barth has noted above, the children usually do not fit neatly into certain categories as do many other special-needs children, such as those who are clearly developmentally delayed, physically handicapped, medically fragile, or severely emotionally disturbed. Even for children who do fit into clear-cut categories, studies have shown that adoptive parents often report many unmet service needs (with two of the most commonly cited services being special education and counseling for children), either because services are unavailable or because they are difficult to access [Nelson 1985].

The scarcity of appropriate programs and services for children with prenatal substance exposure has various causes, some related to funding problems and cutbacks. Others stem from the desire—appropriately—to avoid labeling and thereby stigmatizing the children, although the resulting downside is that services do not get tailored to meet these children's needs. In addition, many existing special education and developmental disability systems have been mandated to provide services only for children who have identified developmental delays (including cognitive, physical/motor, communication, or social/emotional impairments), hearing or vision impairments, or a specified combination of factors that place them at high risk for developmental delay. The majority of preschool-aged children with prenatal substance exposure do not fit into these categories. Compounding the problems caused by the paucity of services, the existing standardized, externally structured developmental testing protocols do not readily identify some of these children's vulnerabilities. Some problems—including subtle behavioral deficits and developmental disorganization—may not receive attention even when intervention services are readily available [Beckwith et al. 1994]. When particular deficits are identified, it is often difficult to find helping professionals who are sufficiently knowledgeable, skilled, available, and affordable. Moreover, many of the pertinent service systems that adoptive parents need to access for their children are complex and bureaucratic--school systems, large health care organizations, and agencies that provide services for children with developmental disabilities. These systems can be frustrating to negotiate under the best of circumstances, and maddening when children do not fit neatly into ready categories. The case vignettes on the following pages illustrate how important it is for adoptive parents to advocate actively for services.

Confronting such challenges is not a task for the timid; it is a task for those with a good measure of perseverance and hope.

Confidence in the Usefulness of Intervention

While resiliency and change are always possible for the child and for the adult, resiliency cannot be taken for granted. [Howard et al. 1989: 12]

Tied into the adoptive parents' ability to advocate assertively for services must be a belief in the importance of timely identification of problems, and in the helpfulness of early intervention and services. As noted earlier, researchers agree that exposure of the developing fetus to alcohol or illegal drugs at any time can be detrimental to some degree, that a great deal of neurological development takes place postnatally, and that the range of outcomes for children exposed prenatally to alcohol and/or other drugs may depend on the complex and dynamic interaction between a child's biological vulnerability and aspects of his or her social environment [Barth 1991; Beckwith 1990; Howard et al. 1989; Myers et al. 1992; Tyler 1992; Quinton et al. 1992]. If there is one other tenet to which researchers and clinicians collectively ascribe in this often polarized field, it is

Case Vignette

The adoptive mother of a six-year-old boy with prenatal drug exposure who had been placed with her as a foster child at birth provided every opportunity for this child to achieve his potential and develop good feelings about himself. She brought him for regular developmental evaluations. When he was two years old and feeling frustrated by a speech delay and communication problems, the foster mother sought and obtained speech therapy. With the use of a few signs learned in therapy, the child was able to communicate well enough for his tantrums to diminish. Maturation, ongoing speech therapy, and participation in an enriched preschool program improved his speech. When he was ready to enter first grade, the public school classroom had too many children to permit sufficient attention to his special learning needs, and his adoptive parents located a private school with smaller classrooms and teachers who were able to take the time to individualize the child's program. Thanks to this important change, the boy made many friends and is now enjoying school.

that these children need careful, expert developmental evaluation and follow-up services (at least through their preschool years) to reduce or prevent developmental delays and/or problems with self-regulation and organization, to deal with these difficulties if they do appear, to promote a secure attachment between the children and their caregivers, and to build on the children's potential strengths [Chasnoff 1992; Healey 1993; Howard et al. 1989; Quinton et al. 1992].

All children benefit from the everyday structure and consistency of the home environment to help them establish routines, rituals, and the concept of consequences. These elements of structure can help mitigate the problems related to self-regulatory behavior and disorganization with which many substance-affected children struggle [Rodning et al. 1989]. Should these types of problem behaviors become manifest, however, despite a well-organized caregiving environment, it is important that adoptive parents not personalize them, view them as an embarrassment or a reflection on themselves

Case Vignette

The adoptive mother of a one-year-old girl with prenatal cocaine exposure felt she had received little information and guidance regarding what to expect and how to be helpful to her daughter. She consulted her pediatrician, who admitted that he was not knowledgeable in this area, and then she wrote several letters to experts and centers across the country to gather information and learn how to obtain the assistance and guidance she felt she needed.

or their parenting abilities, or assume that nothing can be done to remedy the situation. Instead, parents must become familiar with early intervention programs, resources, and techniques that exist to promote their children's ability to organize their nervous systems at an early age. In this way, parents can help prevent the establishment of potentially enduring maladaptive compensating patterns of behavior that bring children negative feedback over the long term [Healey 1993].

Because some of the effects of prenatal drug exposure may not become apparent for years, adoptive parents must also be diligent about continuing this follow-up regimen, regarding it not as superfluous or intrusive but as preventive, educational, and helpful anticipatory guidance. If difficulties arise, adoptive parents must be willing to make time to advocate for and access needed services in behalf of their children as well as for themselves. These services might include speech therapy, counseling, enriched preschool programs, special education, respite care, behavior modification, and/or medical services. The need for services should be based less on the confirmation of prenatal drug exposure than on a careful assessment of the individual child's current level of functioning and needs. Parents may need to meet regularly with a variety of professionals from different disciplines, and to establish strong working partnerships with their children's teachers and schools [Tyler 1992]. They must be able and willing to draw upon all available resources when indicated—including family, friends, community networks, professionals, and support groups. While still being respectful of the children, adoptive parents need to be open about the special challenges and problems they face in rearing their children if they are to access the expertise, support, and resulting synergy that can benefit themselves as well as their children. Being very private, feeling that one can take care of things alone, and not having the willingness, fortitude, patience, and time to search out and use systems, supports, and resources can create definite stumbling blocks to obtaining vital help for children and their parents.

Promoting Children's Self-Knowledge and Self-Esteem

In adoption, birth parents are phantom members of the family. The child needs to make this person real, with appropriate characteristics relative to the child's developmental stage...The data seem to indicate that adoptees have room for several parental images that frame who they are. [Cambell et al. 1991: 334]

Approaching adoption with an emphasis on protective factors includes handling children's adoptive status in ways that promote their healthy self-knowledge and self-esteem. Adoptive parents should inform their children openly and positively about the adoption, beginning early enough during the preschool years to ensure that the children first hear this information from their adoptive parents, in a caring way, rather than from others. Furthermore, adoptive parents should use a gradational approach in communicating with their children, in accordance with the way children develop. Research has shown that children's cognitive limitations preclude them from understanding the meaning of adoption until they reach five to seven years of age; until this age range, adopted children tend to show little distress when informed about their status. During the preschool years, children generally understand adoption more in terms of their having been incorporated into their adoptive families, and less in terms of their not having been raised by their biological parents [Brodzinsky 1990]. This is especially true for children who were adopted at birth or shortly afterwards, and who have not experienced re-placements.

What should be conveyed to children during these early years is an attitude of acceptance and affirmation of the adoption, and a recognition that the children's biological origins are human and understandable. The most important messages and attitudes for adoptive parents to communicate during infancy and early childhood are that they feel happy that they adopted their children and that they do not feel opposed to, competitive toward, or insecure about the children's biological parents, or about the children's interest in their biological families or their backgrounds [Dorner 1991]. During a child's very early years, it is seldom necessary to discuss the child's background or a biological parent's substance abuse in any depth because of the child's limited capacity for language and abstraction at this developmental stage. (An important exception, however, would be that of a preschooler who has lived with a substance-abusing family and/or experienced the losses inherent in moving from one home to another.) Adoptive parents should be encouraged to engage in all of the customary family-building and attachment-promoting activities, while recognizing that later on, beginning in the elementary school years, their children are likely to view adoption in a different way and will probably need a fuller explanation about the circumstances of their adoptive placement than they did as preschoolers.

By the time they reach school age, children generally begin to realize that adoption involves loss as well as family-building. With the expansion of cognitive abilities during their school years and adolescence, children begin to realize that they have lost not only their biological parents, but also their sense of connectedness with their ancestry and genealogical history [Brodzinsky 1990; Kirk 1985]. At this point, children who have been adopted often have a strong curiosity about their backgrounds and a desire to understand, express, and integrate their losses. Most adopted children will ask questions if they feel that there is openness and receptivity to their feelings and concerns, and if they are not worried about causing pain to their adoptive parents.

By and large, school-age children and adolescents are developmentally ready to be told what is known about their backgrounds and origins. When parental histories, even those fraught with great struggles and pain, are conveyed in a sensitive, empathic, factual, and nonjudgmental way to children, they can start putting together the gaps in their identity [Dorner 1991]. Children who are helped to do this will be less likely to engage in excessive fantasizing about their backgrounds, and adolescents will be less likely to act to out in an effort to fill in these gaps, compared to those not receiving such information [Sorosky et al. 1978].

In talking with children about prenatal alcohol and/or other drug abuse and the role this problem played in the biological parents' inability to raise them—as in talking with them about any other problems they might be experiencing—honesty, thoughtfulness, and balance are essential. This parallels what Benson and colleagues described as the ideal style for communicating about adoption in general—"a quiet or gentle openness" [Benson et al. 1994: 52]. Combining and integrating the theories and language of Kirk and, later, Brodzinsky, with their own research, Benson and colleagues proposed that "acceptance of child's difference" by adoptive parents promotes their children's mental health, while "denial of child's difference" or "insistence on child's difference" interferes with healthy adjustment [Benson et al. 1994: 57]. Adoptive parents who take this approach provide an environment of acceptance and ease for talking about adoption, initiate conversations about the subject from time to time, and are receptive to discussing the subject when the children bring it up, but do not dwell on it.

Although society, families, and the field of adoption itself have changed greatly since Kirk wrote *Shared Fate* in 1984, his discussion of out-of-wedlock birth as a central issue in a child's background, adoptive parents' feelings about the biological parents' marital status, and ways of sharing this information with children is remarkably applicable to today's situations involving biological parents who abuse alcohol and/or other drugs. Kirk writes about the difficulty adoptive parents often have in accepting the out-of-wedlock beginnings of their children, and about their fear that revealing this information might constitute a problem too overwhelming for a child to handle. Kirk also cites studies, though, indicating that, for adopted persons, out-of-wedlock birth is a more readily acceptable reason for parents to have given up a child than other reasons that might be behind the relinquishment of a child born to a married couple.

Similarly, both adopted children and adults may readily accept that biological parents with chronic substance abuse problems give their children up for adoption because they are unable to care for them. The struggles of chemical dependency are well known in our society and have been well publicized, from cases involving famous athletes to media personalities to the spouses and children of political leaders to the average person on the street. In addition, school-based programs abound to educate children about the problems and long-term impact of alcohol and other drug abuse. Children with prenatal substance exposure might conceivably be clearer about why their biological parents were unable to rear them than if their parents had not had this problem. As Kirk stresses in *Shared Fate*, however, to broach the topic of out-of-wedlock birth with their children in a helpful way, adoptive parents must first sort out their own feelings and attitudes about this subject. This concept is remarkably relevant today for adoptive parents who need to work through their own feelings about biological parents who are chemically dependent, and then share the biological parents' history with their children in an empathic way.

Kirk also notes that, despite universal reproductive norms about children being born into families in which there are both mothers and fathers to receive the newborns, a variety of social conditions may induce people to break with these norms, including unequal access to services and opportunities. Likewise, although reproductive norms in general ordain that a healthy, drug-free pregnancy be promoted, societal and personal circumstances that reduce opportunities, restrict access to resources, and limit choices may be factors that contribute to an individual's violation of this norm by using drugs in general, and during pregnancy in particular. Gender and racial discrimination, poverty, unemployment, inadequate housing, random violence, lack of understanding about the etiology and treatment of chemical dependency, and insufficient resources are just some of these societal conditions. Personal and family experiences in the background of the biological parents—including child abuse, domestic violence, parental addiction, and major losses—are, unfortunately, common among chemically dependent individuals [Edelstein & Kropenske 1992].

By stressing such conditions and the necessity of changing certain social institutions rather than placing blame, adoptive parents can help children with prenatal substance exposure come to terms with the circumstances surrounding their birth. In taking such an approach, adoptive parents do not imply that they view themselves as morally superior to the biological parents, or that they view themselves as having rescued the child. When adoptive parents are able to stress the biological parents' humanness and strengths, when the biological parents are accepted rather than condemned, and when the difficult social situations confronting the biological parents are stressed, adopted children will be less likely to feel compelled to repeat the pattern of chemical dependency manifested by their biological parents; such an acting-out of a self-fulfilling prophesy is more likely to occur when biological parents are devalued and blamed.

Preventing Substance Abuse Problems

Predisposition does not mean predestination. [Schukit 1994: 49]

Substance abuse is a serious problem facing our adolescent population today. In 1993, an estimated 13.6% of all adolescents from 12 to 17 years of age (close to three million young persons) used an illicit drug during the past year, while 35.2% of adolescents (close to 7.5 million youths) had used alcohol during this same period [Substance Abuse and Mental Health Services Administration 1994]. Given these statistics, all children and adolescents are at risk for problems related to alcohol and/or other drug abuse, and youths who were exposed prenatally to drugs may indeed be at increased risk for such problems—although here, once again, it is important to remember that biological and environmental factors are difficult to disentangle. After reviewing the relevant literature and research, Bays [1990: 897] concluded that "children of chemically dependent parents are biologically vulnerable and at increased risk of becoming chemically dependent," although the environment may play a role in increasing or decreasing this risk. Cadoret [1990] likewise concluded that there appears to be a genetic element in alcohol abuse, and possibly in drug abuse as well. The Child Welfare League of America [1992] has cited placement in out-of-home care as a risk factor for developing substance abuse problems because of the loss and stresses that placement involves for the child, no matter how necessary the placement and how nurturing the foster and adoptive caregivers may be. Thus, adoptive parents should keep in mind the value of helping their children develop healthy strategies for coping with feelings of loss and stress in order to prevent children's possible "self-medication" to alleviate painful feelings.

Adoptive parents can work to prevent problems with substance abuse by their child by openly discussing the child's high risk for alcohol and/or other drug abuse problems, and by preparing themselves as well as the child to meet this challenge in the most effective ways available. Here, once again, a delicate balance is essential. Too little discussion and emphasis, on the one hand, can mean that these critical issues remain unexplored and unexpressed, leaving children feeling separated from their adoptive parents and lacking needed guidance, direction, and support. This approach can render children or adolescents unprepared to cope with—and defend against—what might be a predisposition for difficulties with alcohol and/or other drugs. Too much emphasis and insistence, on the other hand, may be intrusive and promote in the children a feeling of being stigmatized and predetermined to experience problems related to substance abuse. This approach also can undermine children's development of confidence in their own abilities, which is central to preventing alcohol and other drug abuse.

A number of excellent and accessible substance abuse prevention curricula targeting children and families as early as the preschool years are available (e.g., Getting a Head Start Against Drugs, coauthored by the National Head Start Association and the Center for Substance Abuse Prevention [Carter & Oyemaded 1993]). Adoptive parents of children with prenatal substance exposure can benefit from involving themselves and their children in programs that use such constructive approaches, particularly because the principles presented in such curricula are basically health-building, long-term approaches for enhancing effective parenting and strengthening all families. These principles include focusing on the strengths of each family member, identifying and developing activities that make every person feel good naturally, developing self-esteem in all family members, learning to cope with anger and stress, and enhancing communication skills. Also emphasized is the importance of helping children understand that there are no quick fixes, but instead teaching them to value perseverance and honest effort. Educating oneself and one's children to be aware of the realities, signs, effects, and dangers associated with substance abuse problems, maintaining clear rules and expectations about the use of alcohol and other drugs by children, and setting appropriate parental examples are other critical elements in any substance abuse prevention program. Contributing to and drawing upon support from family, friends, and the community are also vital to such an approach [Carter & Oyemaded 1993]. If substance abuse-related problems do arise, understanding the importance of intervening early and effectively, and having the willingness and ability to access necessary services are crucial and may even be lifesaving.

Children must be made aware that they have the power and control to make decisions and choices regarding substance abuse. Parents hold the key to this awareness. They must take the additional step of teaching children to assume personal responsibility by considering the impact of their actions on themselves as well as others. For an individual who is armed with information, strategies, and healthy coping skills, a predisposition to substance abuse can remain just that. It does not have to materialize into a problem.

Summary

In contemplating adoption of a child with prenatal substance exposure, prospective adoptive parents should give much thought to their hopes and expectations for the child they will be adopting. These initial hopes and expectations should be balanced, however, by what the child brings to the family—his or her own unique array of strengths, vulnerabilities, and needs. The adoptive parents will have to be flexible enough to adapt to the child as she or he grows and changes over the years. As adopted children develop and gain additional understanding about the meaning of adoption, they will confront the same issues regarding their origins, losses, and uncertainties that their adoptive parents have had to come to terms with. If, throughout this process, adoptive parents are able to empathize with their children's biological parents, the children ultimately will incorporate this compassion into their own feelings of self-worth.

Adoptive applicants will likely find that, in some situations, they should become advocates for their children, not only to ensure that the children receive needed services, but also to provide their children with every opportunity to succeed. This will require time and effort as parents learn to navigate systems that may not be familiar to them. Networking with informed professionals and other parents in similar circumstances can open the door for adoptive parents to locate the most useful resources available.

Finally, with regard to future dangers for all children, and perhaps especially for children with prenatal substance exposure, honest communication with children and instilling in children an appreciation of the value of a healthy life-style are the essence of substance abuse prevention.

References

Barth, R. P. (1991). Adoption of drug-exposed children. *Children and Youth Services Review, 13*, 323–342.

Bays, J. (1990). Substance abuse and child abuse: Impact of addiction on the child. *Pediatric Clinics of North America, 37*, 881–904.

Beckwith, L. (1990). Adaptive and maladaptive parenting: Implications for intervention. In S. Meisels and J. Shankoff (Eds.), *Handbook of early childhood intervention* (pp. 53–77). New York: Cambridge University Press.

Beckwith, L., Rodning, C., Norris, D., Phillipsen, L., Khandabi, P., & Howard, J. (1994). Spontaneous play in two-year-olds born to substance-abusing mothers. *Infant Mental Health Journal, 15*, 189–201.

Benson, P. L., Sharma, A. R., & Roehlkepartain, E. C. (1994). *Growing up adopted: A portrait of adolescents and their families.* Minneapolis, MN: Search Institute.

Brodzinsky, D. M. (1990). A stress and coping model of adoption adjustment. In D. M. Brodzinsky & M. D. Schechter (Eds.), *The psychology of adoption* (2nd ed.) (pp. 3–24). New York: Oxford University Press.

Brown, S. L. (1992). Fetal alcohol syndrome research. *The Roundtable: Journal of the National Resource Center for Special Needs Adoption, 6*(2), 5–7.

Cadoret, R. J. (1990). Biologic perspectives of adoptee adjustment. In D. M. Brodzinsky & M. D. Schechter (Eds.), *The psychology of adoption* (2nd ed.) (pp. 25–41). New York: Oxford University Press.

Cambell, L. H., Silverman, P. R., & Patti, P. B. (1991). Reunions between adoptees and birthparents: The adoptee's experience. *Social Work, 36*, 329–335.

Carter, S., & Oyemaded, U. J. (1993). *Getting a head start against drugs.* Washington, DC: U.S. Department of Health and Human Services, Public Health Service, Substance Abuse and Mental Health Services Administration, National Head Start Association and Center for Substance Abuse Prevention.

Chasnoff, I. J. (1992, August). Cocaine, pregnancy, and the growing child. *Current Problems in Pediatrics,* 302–321.

Child Welfare League of America. (1992). *Children at the front: A different view of the war on alcohol and drugs. Final report of the CWLA North American Commission on Chemical Dependency and Child Welfare.* Washington, DC: Author.

Dorner, P. M. (1991). *Talking to your child about adoption.* Mt. Herman, CA: Schaeffer Publishing Company.

Edelstein, S. B., & Kropenske, V. (1992). Assessment and psychosocial issues for drug-dependent women. In M. Jessup (Ed.), *Drug dependency in pregnancy: Managing withdrawal* (pp. 13–36). North Highlands, CA: California Department of Health Services, Maternal and Child Health Branch (State of California, Department of General Services, Publication Section).

Fink, J. R. (1992). Advocacy on behalf of drug-exposed children: Legal perspectives. In S. L. Quinton, S. A. Johnson, E. M. Johnson, R. W. Denniston, & K. L. Augustson (Eds.), *Identifying the needs of drug-affected children: Public policy issues* (pp. 139–150). Rockville, MD: Office for Substance Abuse Prevention; U.S. Department of Health and Human Services (OSAP prevention monograph 11, DHHS publication number ADM 92–1814).

Healey, T. (1993). Intervention strategies in children prenatally exposed to drugs... a continuum birth through school age. *The Clearinghouse for Drug Exposed Children Newsletter,* 4(3), 1–3, 6.

Howard, J., Beckwith, L., Rodning, C., & Kropenske, V. (1989). The development of young children of substance-abusing parents: Insights from seven years of intervention and research. *Zero to Three,* 9(5), 8–12.

Kirk, H. D. (1985). *Adoptive kinship: A modern institution in need of reform.* Port Angeles, WA: Ben-Simon Publications.

McGuire, A. (1983). My child was born today. In P. I. Johnston (Ed.), *Perspectives on a grafted tree: Thoughts for those touched by adoption* (p. 39). Indianapolis, IN: Perspectives Press.

Miller, N. B. (1994). *Nobody's perfect.* Baltimore: Paul H. Brookes Publishing Company.

Myers, B. J., Olson, H. C., & Kaltenbach, K. (1992). Cocaine-exposed infants: Myths and misunderstandings. *Zero to Three, 13*(1), 1–5.

Nelson, K. A. (1985). *On the frontier of adoption: A study of special-needs adoptive families.* New York: Child Welfare League of America, Inc.

Quinton, S. L., Johnson, S. A., Johnson, E. M., Denniston, R. W., & Augustson K. L. (Eds.) (1992). Introduction. In *Identifying the needs of drug-affected children: Public policy issues* (pp. 1–10). Rockville, MD: Office for Substance Abuse Prevention; U.S. Department of Health and Human Services (OSAP prevention monograph 11, DHHS publication number ADM 92–1814).

Rodning, C., Beckwith, L., & Howard, J. (1989). Characteristics of attachment organization and play organization in prenatally drug-exposed toddlers. *Development and Psychopathology, 1,* 277–289.

Rosenthal, J. A., & Groze, V. K. (1992). *Special-needs adoption: A study of intact families.* New York: Praeger Publishers.

Rosenthal, J. A. (1993, Spring). Outcomes of adoption of children with special needs. *The Future of Children, 3*(1), 83, 77–88.

Schukit, M. (1994). Addiction: A whole new view. *Psychology Today, 27*(5), 49.

Severson, R. W. (1991). *Adoption: Charms and rituals for healing.* Dallas, TX: House of Tomorrow Productions.

Silverstein, D., & Kaplan, S. (1989). Seven core issues in adoption: A therapeutic framework. In L. Coleman, K. Tibor, H. Hornby, & C. Boggis (Eds.), *Working with older adoptees.* Tustin, CA: Parenting Resources.

Sorosky, A. D., Baran, A., & Pannor, R. (1978). *The adoption triangle.* Garden City, NY: Anchor Press/Doubleday. (Anchor Books Edition 1984).

Substance Abuse and Mental Health Services Administration, Office of Applied Studies (1994, October). *National household survey on drug abuse: Population estimates 1993.* Rockville, MD: U.S. Department of Health and Human Services, Public Health Service (DHHS Publication number SMA 94–3017).

Tyler, R. (1992, May). Prenatal drug exposure: An overview of associated problems and intervention strategies. *Phi Delta Kappan, 73,* 705–708.

Weiss, E. (1989). *Mothers talk about learning disabilities: Personal feelings, practical advice.* New York: Prentice Hall Press.

Young, N. K., Wallace, V. R., & Garcia, T. (1992, Spring). Developmental status of three to five year-old children who were prenatally exposed to alcohol and other drugs. *School Social Work Journal, 16,* 1–15.

V

Recommendations

Children have only one childhood. If that childhood consists of regular, constant, reliable, loving relationships, it is likely that the child will develop a sense of belonging, a necessary ingredient for good citizenship as an adult. If those conditions do not exist, then the child's future may well be in doubt. [Walker 1994: 148]

Although this book seeks primarily to highlight relevant clinical considerations for adults who are thinking about adopting a child with prenatal alcohol and/or other drug exposure, a number of recommendations inevitably arise. This chapter highlights some of the most significant of these recommendations, not only to point out directions for future efforts in the field of adoption of children with prenatal substance exposure, but also to provide a context for professionals in their ongoing work with families. Realistic expectations and goals must take into account the characteristics of the individual child, adoptive applicant, and family situation, as well as the larger community and service system environment within which the new family will make its life.

Services for Biological Parents Who Abuse Alcohol and/or Other Drugs

Recommendations related to the adoption of children with prenatal substance exposure must begin with the biological parents—the initial members of the adoption triangle, without whom there would be no adoption process to consider. Largely due to the persistent and pervasive nature of problems related to chemical dependency, the needs of substance-abusing biological parents are vast.

Pre- and Postadoption Counseling

Biological parents who are pregnant and are considering adoption as a possible option for their children should have access to adoption professionals who have a sufficient level of expertise regarding chemical dependency. To be helpful to such parents, practitioners must be knowledgeable about the psychosocial elements of alcoholism and addiction; the range of legal, emotional, social, and medical problems commonly experienced by individuals who abuse substances; and the impact of alcohol and other drug dependency on pregnancy, parenting, and individual and family functioning. Professionals must be familiar with techniques for interviewing and developing rapport with substance-abusing clients, and able to feel comfortable discussing the various aspects of alcohol and other drug use and the chemically dependent life-style. Professionals must also be aware that an individual who has problems related to substance abuse may also have a primary psychiatric disorder; thus, a familiarity with strategies for working with persons who are "dual diagnosed" is helpful. Professionals must understand the importance of—and be able to advocate for—coordinated and comprehensive substance abuse treatment and prenatal care, and emphasize in their work with clients the consequences of not seeking or following through with these services. They also should be skilled in helping biological parents express their full range of feelings, hopes, and fears about their unborn child [Edelstein & Kropenske 1992].

Effective counselors must be able to encourage all parents (usually the biological mother) to explore thoroughly and in a timely fashion all options for the pregnancy, including supported childbirth and child-rearing, kinship or family foster care, adoption, or termination of pregnancy [Edelstein & Kropenske 1992]. If adoption is the choice, professionals have to be able to explain the different types of adoption, and make themselves available before, during, and following relinquishment and placement to assist with support and counseling. Postrelinquishment availability is particularly important for substance-dependent parents because their abuse of alcohol and/or other drugs may have been a coping mechanism for dealing with previous losses. Parents may be especially vulnerable at this time and in need of support, grief counseling, encouragement, and coordination of services if they are to emerge from this crisis in an adaptive way, with plans for their children that they can live with, and with healthier ways of coping with problems and losses in their lives.

Guidelines and Services to Support Family Preservation

In situations in which parents are chemically dependent and their children have been exposed prenatally to alcohol and/or other drugs, but in which the children's safety has not been compromised to the extent that out-of-home placement has been deemed necessary, every effort should be made at the outset to explore ways for maintaining the family and enhancing the biological parent-child relationship. A number of important conditions, however, must be present to successfully maintain children in families with chemically dependent parents. First, the biological parents must be committed to keeping their family together as well as to acting in ways that will help make this desire a reality. For some parents, chemical dependency is so powerful and all-consuming a drive that both the desire and the ability to parent may be obliterated. Second, to make family preservation efforts successful, the biological parents must be willing and able to use appropriate resources (e.g., substance abuse treatment and parenting education programs) to break through their chemical dependency and reduce the risks to their children [Child Welfare League of America 1992]. Third, the biological parents must be able to engage consistently and effectively with these services within a time-frame that is appropriate for their children's development.

Guidelines and Services to Support Family Reunification

In some situations in which parents are chemically dependent, the risks of child abuse and/or neglect may be too great to keep families together, despite the best efforts of helping professionals. In such cases, out-of-home placement may be necessary. As Goldstein and colleagues [1979: 5, 6] stated in their classic, *Before the Best Interests of the Child*, however, "The goal of intervention must be to create or recreate a family for the child as quickly as possible," and "Placement decisions should reflect the child's, not the adult's, sense of time."

Although denial is a predictable element of chemical dependency, as is the inevitable possibility of relapse, the crisis created by the removal of a child can serve as the impetus for parents to acknowledge a problem and engage in treatment—even if it is the first of several attempts at sobriety/abstinence. For substance-affected families, the course of reunification will almost always take longer than it would for nonaffected families because of the tenacious and chronic nature of chemical dependency. Nevertheless, children cannot wait for parents who are not available to them or to child protective services workers. Parents have to be present and actively involved in rehabilitation.

For substance-affected parents to engage effectively and in a timely way with useful services, however, the services must be available and accessible, without extensive waiting lists. This must be the case for parents who are seeking these services voluntarily during the prenatal period, as well as for parents who have been involuntarily mandated to do so following their children's birth. Furthermore, within child protective services agencies, child welfare workers must have manageable caseloads to be able to assess and assist these complex families from the very beginning, and to provide the intensive and long-term services they almost invariably require [Child Welfare League of America 1992].

Guidelines for Termination of Parental Rights

Failure to make early decisions and a lack of aggressive adoptive planning frequently cause children to languish in the system. [Walker 1994: 149]

In some cases, substance abuse may have weakened already vulnerable parents to the point where it is no longer in the children's best interests to be with them. In such instances, there must be a clear delineation of the point at which children are entitled to a permanent home apart from their biological families. Thus, the child welfare system must work together with the substance abuse treatment, legal, and political arenas to meet the needs of chemically dependent families and also to decide on the point at which permanent plans should be made [Child Welfare League of America 1992].

Additionally, in situations involving substance-affected parents and relatives who are absent and thus unavailable to engage in planning, case reviews and permanency planning should be expedited. Under circumstances where early and thorough assessments point to the unlikelihood of family reunification, involved practitioners must be aware that infants and children who were exposed prenatally to alcohol and/or other drugs may be biologically at risk and therefore in need of stable, permanent, and sensitive placement as early as possible in order to reduce environmental risks. The importance of early adoptive placement has long been established and cannot be overemphasized. Promoting early positive attachments and optimizing the environment can be decisive factors for some of the prenatally substance-exposed children's long-term outcomes. Perhaps priority can be given to the earliest possible permanent placement for children with prenatal drug exposure. If such a placement is not achievable with relatives, the children need to be placed as early as possible with nonrelated adoptive parents who have been thoroughly and appropriately prepared. If parental rights to the child are *likely* but not certain to be terminated, and determination will require an extended period of time, efforts should be made to place the young child with foster parents who are prepared to adopt if parental rights should be terminated, but who also fully understand the legal and emotional risks involved in such a placement and can accept and fulfill the role of foster parents as well. In current practice, bureaucratic constraints frequently hinder creative options; excessive caution, large caseloads, limited resources, lack of awareness, and/or lack of communication among child welfare workers performing various functions also impede such placements.

Wald [1994] notes that obstacles to providing permanent homes for children in situations involving parental chemical dependency appear to be related to agency and court practices rather than to statutory concerns, since most states have applicable laws for termination of parental rights. He goes on to say that immediate termination of parental rights should be considered if the custodial parent is unable to provide regular care for the child and refuses appropriate treatment services. When reunification is not possible, termination of parental rights followed as quickly as possible by adoptive placement is preferable to legal guardianship, especially for young children, as adoption affords the child increased stability and additional opportunities to experience the positive commitment of adults. Termination of parental rights generally should be seriously considered for children under age three who are not well on their way toward reunification with their biological parents within one year of placement in out-of-home care.

It is not uncommon for infants and young children to be placed initially in foster homes without regard to the appropriateness of the home for long-term placement, even when family reunification is unlikely. Later, when time frames for considering termination of parental rights are finally reached, and the foster family is unable or unwilling to adopt, parental rights are often not terminated because of the wish to avoid severing the emotional ties that develop between the foster parent and the child. In such cases, the child is not afforded the permanency of adoption, but instead is provided with an alternative that offers a reduced likelihood of a lifetime commitment.

Additionally, even though it is best for foster family placements overall to be made with parents of the same race and culture as the child [Child Welfare League of America 1992], this too does not always occur. If the foster parents are of a different race and culture from the child, despite all good intentions, in some cases they may not be sensitive to or capable of meeting the special challenges of a transracial/transcultural placement or the unique long-term needs of the child.

In these situations, careful, timely, and creative planning often can provide more suitable and permanent long-term plans. One alternative, for example, might be to actively and concurrently pursue and evaluate permanent placement possibilities while providing the biological parents with additional time and resources to support rehabilitation. Within this option, if it is decided that parental rights will be terminated, the necessary and time-consuming home studies will have been completed, obviating further delays in achieving permanency for the child.

Services for Adoptive Parents

If children with prenatal substance exposure who cannot be maintained with their own biological or extended families are to have permanent families by adoption, significant efforts must be put into recruiting, educating, and preparing adoptive parents for these children, as well as providing these families and their children with substantive postplacement services. Because child welfare agencies have the greatest potential to deliver a range of critical services to biological parents as well as to adoptive parents and children, their involvement in the adoption of children with prenatal drug exposure would seem most appropriate.

Recruitment

Before recruiting adoptive parents for children with prenatal alcohol and/or other drug exposure, recruiters need to be sure that their personal feelings, attitudes, and beliefs about alcoholism/addiction do not interfere with their task. Recruiters must also know enough about the special considerations involved in adopting children who were prenatally substance-exposed to ensure that their presentations and responses to inquiries are informed. Ideally, representatives of all of the various disciplines involved in working with substance-affected families would participate in recruitment efforts in order to respond effectively to the questions raised by prospective adoptive applicants. These disciplines should include social services, medicine, nursing, education, substance abuse treatment, child development, and psychology. Furthermore, it is of major importance that efforts be made to recruit adoptive parents from each child's race and culture. Finally, the essence of the recruitment message should be that prenatal substance exposure is a risk factor, but that with adequate preparation and supports, this risk is very much worth taking for many families and individuals.

Educational and Preparative Services

> Social workers must dispel the belief of many adoptive families that love and a positive environment will resolve all problems and must provide counseling services to help deal with the problems that may arise. [Grotevant & McRoy 1990: 185]

It is essential that prospective adoptive parents are thoroughly educated and prepared regarding what the adoption of an infant or child with prenatal substance exposure might involve—including the joys, risks, possibilities, and extent of the challenge if risks materialize into realities and problems have to be managed. Time and time again, research has shown that the better the preparation, the more satisfied the adoptive parents are with the adoption. Thorough preparation (through access to up-to-date information) allows adoptive parents to play an active role, make informed decisions, and thus feel in control. Although most prospective adoptive parents do not initially request an infant or child with prenatal substance exposure, stretching preferences to include such a child might well be appropriate as long as the adoptive applicants are fully prepared and willingly make an informed decision that this kind of placement is right for them. It should also be noted that minor impairments in a child (such as learning disabilities or developmental delays) often pose more problems for adoptive parents than multiple major developmental impairments, and that minor impairments can be correlated with more negative adoption outcomes. Often, adoptive parents are better prepared for major impairments than minor ones because the former are usually readily noticed and diagnosed, while minor problems may catch unprepared adoptive parents unawares [Rosenthal & Groze 1992]. In addition, as compared to their view of major impairments, adoptive parents are more likely to view minor impairments with unrealistic optimism [Rosenthal 1993], which can convert to future disappointment in the child if the optimism proves unwarranted. Subtle, minor impairments are common among infants and children with prenatal drug exposure; they highlight the need for thorough preparation of adoptive applicants in order to prevent disappointment with an adopted child who has been exposed prenatally to alcohol and/or other drugs.

Thorough preparation involves time, reinforcement, and ongoing assessment and discussion with prospective adoptive parents about their feelings and concerns. Reinforcement is necessary because many adoptive applicants have difficulty understanding and incorporating information due to anxiety, inexperience, fearfulness about being rejected by the agency, and/or extreme or even desperate eagerness to have a child [Nelson 1985]. In addition, the issues and emotions concerning chemically dependent biological parents and children with prenatal alcohol and/or other drug exposure are indeed complex.

The process of education/preparation, exploration, and assessment should be conducted with each individual applicant, and jointly with couples, according to the family constellation. Applicant groups–small or large, depending upon the clients' needs—can also be extremely helpful settings in which to learn, explore, and contribute. Again, group education is best conducted by an interdisciplinary team that includes some combination of social workers, physicians, nurses, child development specialists, educators, psychologists, substance abuse treatment counselors, experienced adoptive parents who have adopted children with prenatal substance exposure, and perhaps also substance abusers in recovery. This approach provides extensive preparation and has proven to be effective in helping applicants, who, deciding that adopting a child who may have special needs is not for them, self-select out of the process. This approach also models teamwork and the benefits of consultation and collaboration, elements that may turn out to be important to the families at some later point. Suggested topics to be covered in the education/preparation and discussion groups include:

- Attitudes, feelings, and beliefs about chemical dependency in general, and about substance abuse during pregnancy in particular;

- Substances of abuse and adult chemical dependence;

- Psychosocial dynamics of parental substance abuse;

- Normal child development;

- Medical and neurobehavioral concerns for children with prenatal substance exposure;

- Development of infants and children who were exposed to alcohol and/or other drugs in utero;

- Review of contradictory media accounts and their impact;

- Special issues for adoptive parents of children with prenatal substance exposure (including the special issues described in this book);

- Caregiving strategies for high-risk infants, toddlers, and preschoolers;

- Child care techniques, toys, and play activities that can

benefit infants and children who were exposed prenatally to alcohol and/or other drugs;

- Common satisfactions and stresses experienced by foster and adoptive parents of children with prenatal substance exposure;

- Special issues in transracial adoption;

- Importance of early identification and intervention;

- Skills and expertise of the various professionals who can contribute to the care of prenatally drug-exposed children and their families;

- Community resources and systems for high-risk children and the skills needed to negotiate these systems; and

- Substance abuse prevention.

After receiving this type of preparation, prospective adoptive parents should be in a better position to make informed decisions about whether the adoption of a child with prenatal substance exposure is in their own as well as in the child's best interests. As Nelson wrote in *On the Frontier of Adoption: A Study of Special Needs Adoptive Families*, adoptive parents' educated opinions about the appropriateness of a placement are important predictors of outcome for an adoption [Nelson 1985].

Anticipatory Guidance

When adoptive applicants indicate that they wish to consider placement of a child with prenatal substance exposure and there is a particular child for them to consider, agencies can provide support in several ways throughout the decision-making process. First, agencies should release to the applicants, in writing, all available medical and social history about the biological parents, the child, and the extended family. Attempts also should be made to fill in information gaps, if this is at all possible [Nelson 1985]. According to Rosenthal and Groze [1992], the availability of in-depth information and thorough preparation are especially important for applicants who are stretching their preferences to include children who may have special needs, because these adoptive applicants can be at high risk for feeling dissatisfied or disappointed with the child after placement.

This certainly applies to applicants who come in hoping to adopt an infant without problems and who then decide, generally because of the scarcity of such infants, to consider adopting an infant or toddler who has been exposed prenatally to drugs.

Moreover, professionals should inform adoptive parents not only when there is evidence of prenatal substance exposure, but also when it is reasonable to consider that this is a possibility. For example, if the mother's symptoms or life-style, relatives' or professionals' statements, or the child's condition seem consistent with a history of maternal substance abuse—even when there has been no positive toxicology screen—this possibility should be raised with prospective adoptive parents. Disclosing this information, whether as fact or as likelihood, shows respect for the adoptive applicants, helps them make more informed decisions about whether to proceed with the placement, and contributes to a relationship of trust. Providing this information also helps ensure that the child will receive appropriate medical and developmental assessments that can identify potential problems, thereby ensuring that timely preventive services will be sought [Child Welfare League of America 1992].

An adoption worker once stated to the primary author of this volume that, since the toxicology screen on the infant was negative, he did not consider it necessary or even appropriate to tell the prospective adoptive parents that the infant had been exposed prenatally to drugs, even though the mother had disclosed to this same worker that she used phencyclidine (PCP) throughout pregnancy. Fortunately, the worker was receptive to clarification of the issue and there was time to rectify the situation, but this example demonstrates how important it is for practitioners to be thoroughly prepared for this kind of special-needs adoption work if applicants are to be thoroughly prepared and children's futures safeguarded.

Ongoing Supportive Services

Because some children with prenatal alcohol and/or other drug exposure require specialized care, publicly funded financial assistance and medical coverage may be indicated and should be provided at the time of adoptive placement. For other such children, however, no special care appears necessary initially, and in fact may never be indicated. In some situations, the full extent of the child's needs may not be apparent at the time of placement, and, whenever the child's circumstances and agency regulations permit, there should be a commitment to provide financial and medical assistance to meet real expenses in the future should this become necessary. Knowing that they can return to reevaluate the cost of caring for the child's special needs could help reduce some adoptive applicants' uncertainties and concerns about the future of their children.

In addition, for those children and families who do need such assistance over the years, support, guidance, and advocacy for services are critical and should be available. Families may need help identifying and accessing services and resources such as speech therapy, therapeutic preschool programs, special education programs, developmental assessments, child care, support groups, behavioral management training, transportation, health and mental health care, and professionals skilled in working with children at high risk as well as with the nature of adoption. Support groups that connect new and experienced adoptive parents who have adopted children with prenatal substance exposure can be invaluable sources of helpful strategies and resources, and allow adoptive parents to give and gain support and reduce isolation. As Kirk [1984: 122] has written, "Self-help organizations may add to their members' sense of autonomy...The hazards of the unexplored area can frequently be dealt with best by cooperative action."

These postadoption services have to be available indefinitely, on an as-needed basis, because of changing family needs over time, the challenges that some of these children may present, and the ongoing development of research and strategies that can be shared with families. Workshops and conferences for parents and for professionals should be conducted regularly to review in greater depth the matters discussed in the education/preparation stage.

Cross-Training for Professionals

We've solved most of the easy problems. What we're left with are some very difficult, complex issues, and... the old single-discipline approach is simply not going to work anymore. [Winer 1992: 38]

As noted above, to provide meaningful support for biological and adoptive families in this field, practitioners must be sensitive to and skillful regarding an entire range of concerns related to alcohol and/ or other drug abuse. Overall, professionals should feel comfortable exploring complex and emotionally laden topics, and should be familiar with techniques for interviewing and developing rapport with sometimes challenging clients. They also must be knowledgeable about problems related to alcoholism and addiction and the impact of chemical dependency on individual and family functioning. In addition, they must have some knowledge of the potential effects of prenatal substance exposure on child development. Perhaps most importantly, however, professionals need to be aware of the multiple agencies and professional disciplines that are involved in serving substance-affected families—including child welfare and social services, medicine, nursing, education, child development, psychology, substance abuse treatment, and the legal system—and to recognize the importance of coordinated, interdisciplinary services for substance-affected families. Working with families who are affected by alcohol and/or other drug abuse by necessity involves interagency and interdisciplinary teamwork, as well as skilled assessment and intervention with biological parents, relatives, foster parents, and adoptive parents caring for infants and children with prenatal substance exposure. Thus, training for professionals working in this area is best provided by a team of experts from the fields of medicine, child welfare, nursing, child development, and substance abuse treatment—the disciplines most commonly involved in working with substance-affected families [Edelstein et al. 1990].

Conclusion

If we are to provide the large number of children who have been exposed prenatally to alcohol and/or other drugs with the permanent families many of them desperately need, then appropriate services are necessary for biological parents; for recruiting, educating, and supporting adoptive families; and for adequately preparing service providers to assist these families. If children who were exposed prenatally to alcohol and/or other drugs cannot achieve permanency with their biological parents or in kinship care, then society owes them the security, growth, and opportunity that adoption can provide. We cannot expect families to take on these challenges and responsibilities, however, without the necessary assistance. In the long run, we will all benefit by giving these children every chance to develop their potential and to overcome their difficult beginnings.

References

Child Welfare League of America (1992). *Children at the front: A different view of the war on alcohol and drugs. Final report of the CWLA National Commission on Chemical Dependency and Child Welfare.* Washington, DC: Author.

Edelstein, S. B., & Kropenske, V. (1992). Assessment and psychosocial issues for drug-dependent women. In M. Jessup (Ed.), *Drug dependency in pregnancy: Managing withdrawal* (pp. 13–36). North Highlands, CA: California Department of Health Services, Maternal and Child Health Branch (State of California, Department of General Services, Publication Section).

Edelstein, S. B., Kropenske, V., & Howard, J. (1990). Project T.E.A.M.S. *Social Work, 35,* 313–318.

Goldstein, J., Freud, A., & Solnit, A. J. (1979). *Before the best interests of the child.* New York: The Free Press.

Grotevant, H. D., & McRoy, R. G. (1990). Adopted adolescents in residential treatment: The role of the family. In D. M. Brodzinsky & M. D. Schechter (Eds.), *The psychology of adoption* (2nd ed.) (pp. 167–186). New York: Oxford University Press.

Kirk, H. D. (1984). *Shared fate: A theory and method of adoptive relationships* (2nd ed.). Port Angeles, WA: Ben-Simon Publications.

Nelson, K. A. (1985). *On the frontier of adoption: A study of special needs adoptive families.* New York: Child Welfare League of America, Inc.

Rosenthal, J. A., & Groze, V. K. (1992). *Special-needs adoption: A study of intact families.* New York: Praeger Publishers.

Wald, M. S. (1994). Termination of parental rights. In D. J. Besharov (Ed.), *When drug addicts have children: Reorienting child welfare's response* (pp. 195–210). Washington, DC: Child Welfare League of America, Inc.

Walker, C. D. (1994). African American children in foster care. In D. J. Besharov (Ed.), *When drug addicts have children: Reorienting child welfare's response* (pp. 145–152). Washington, DC: Child Welfare League of America, Inc.

Winer, A. (1992). Quoted in M. Kort (1992). Boundary crossings. *UCLA Magazine, 4*(1), 33-38.

About the Authors

Susan Edelstein is a licensed clinical social worker who has worked with vulnerable children, parents, and families in Los Angeles for over 27 years. She earned her bachelor of arts degree at the University of California, Los Angeles, and her master's degree in Social Welfare at the University of Southern California. Ms. Edelstein began her career in child protective services, then specialized in adoptions for six years, and in 1979 began her work at the UCLA Medical Center as coordinator of the Suspected Child Abuse and Neglect (SCAN) Team. For the past decade, within the Developmental Studies Program, UCLA School of Medicine, she has directed and co-directed several major service, training, and research projects involving inter-disciplinary-interagency collaboration, child abuse and neglect, parental chemical dependency, and comprehensive early intervention approaches. Her work has encompassed collaboration with all of the contributing authors of this book.

In the course of her experience, Ms. Edelstein became aware of the lack of information about children with prenatal substance exposure whose needs for permanency would best be met by adoption, and about the limited guidelines for professionals in preparing and supporting adoptive and prospective adoptive parents of these children. This book grew out of her concern and commitment to presenting these issues in a holistic, balanced, and informed manner, specifically with reference to the preparation of prospective adoptive parents.

Judy Howard is a professor of pediatrics at the UCLA School of Medicine and currently heads the Developmental Studies Program within the UCLA Department of Pediatrics. Dr. Howard has directed the UCLA Intervention Program for Children with Disabilities since 1974 and chaired the UCLA Child Abuse Policy Committee for over a decade. Since 1982, she has been principal investigator on a variety of service, training, and research projects relating to prenatal substance abuse and services for affected children, caregivers, and families. Dr. Howard received her medical degree from the Loma Linda School of Medicine, did her pediatric residency at the Los Angeles County/University of Southern California School of Medicine, and completed subspecialty training in child development at the UCLA Department of Pediatrics.

A developmental pediatrician and assistant professor of pediatrics at UCLA, *Rachelle Tyler* has had extensive clinical and research experience working with substance-affected children and families over the past 12 years. She earned her medical degree at the Boston University School of Medicine, did her pediatric residency at the Martin Luther King, Jr., General Hospital in Los Angeles, and completed subspecialty training in child development at the UCLA School of Pediatrics. In 1982 she earned a master's degree in Public Health, focusing on health services organization, at the UCLA School of Public Health. Dr. Tyler currently directs two pediatric clinics providing developmental assessments and case management services for medically fragile infants, many of whom were exposed prenatally to alcohol and/or other drugs. She also heads an ongoing training program promoting interdisciplinary teamwork among community-based professionals in Los Angeles County serving children who were exposed prenatally to drugs and their caregivers.

Gloria Waldinger's career in child welfare has included direct practice in public child welfare settings, management of a number of federally funded child welfare training grant programs, and administration, teaching, and research at the UCLA School of Social Welfare. The focuses of her direct practice and research have been the adoption of special-needs children, child abuse and neglect, guardianship, and the emancipation of children from out-of-home care. Dr. Waldinger is a recognized expert in child welfare policy and is currently serving as consultant to the Los Angeles County Department of Children and Family Services' Family Preservation and Family Support Program. She also participates actively in community organizations dealing with programs and policies for children and families. She received both her master's and doctoral degrees in Social Welfare at the University of California, Los Angeles.

Annette Moore has worked with the interdisciplinary team of the UCLA Developmental Studies Program since 1988. During this time, she has provided administrative and writing / editorial support on a range of clinical service, research, and training programs related to children and families affected by parental abuse of alcohol and / or other drugs. This work has encompassed collaboration in the preparation of grant proposals, articles, training manuals, and curricula for local, state, and national programs. Her academic background includes a bachelor's degree in English, German, and art from California State University, Sacramento, as well as a master's degree in Germanic languages from the University of California, Los Angeles.